UPDATES AND ADVANCES IN NEPHROLITHIASIS - PATHOPHYSIOLOGY, GENETICS, AND TREATMENT MODALITIES

Edited by **Layron Long**

Updates and Advances in Nephrolithiasis - Pathophysiology, Genetics, and Treatment Modalities
http://dx.doi.org/10.5772/65175
Edited by Layron Long

Contributors

Fay Hill, John Andrew Sayer, Noha Maraie, Omar Mohammed Osman, Hosni Khairy Salem, Rongwei Jason Xuan, Thomas Hasenberg, Jian James Zhang, Giovanna Priante, Federica Quaggio, Liliana Terrin, Monica Ceol, Lisa Gianesello, Dorella Del Prete, Franca Anglani, Onur Kaygısız

Published by InTech
Janeza Trdine 9, 51000 Rijeka, Croatia

Publishing Process Manager Martina Usljebrka
Technical Editor SPi Global
Cover InTech Design team

First published August, 2017
Printed in Croatia
Legal deposit, Croatia: National and University Library in Zagreb

Additional hard copies can be obtained from orders@intechopen.com

Updates and Advances in Nephrolithiasis - Pathophysiology, Genetics, and Treatment Modalities, Edited by Layron Long
p. cm.
Print ISBN 978-953-51-3459-6
Online ISBN 978-953-51-3460-2

For EU product safety concerns:
IN TECH d.o.o., Prolaz Marije Krucifikse Kozulić 3, 51000 Rijeka, Croatia,
info@intechopen.com or visit our website at intechopen.com.

Meet the editor

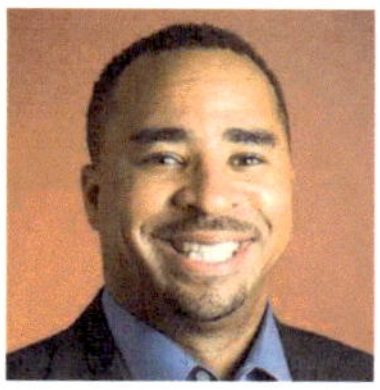

Dr. Long is a board certified urologist who earned a doctorate of medicine from Meharry Medical College in Nashville, TN. He then completed general surgery internship at Vanderbilt University Medical Center in Nashville, TN, and a fellowship in Molecular Genetics at the Howard University/Johns Hopkins University in the Washington DC and Baltimore Maryland.

Dr. Long trained in urological surgery at TUFTS New England Medical Center in Boston, MA, and completed his senior and chief resident years of training at the University of Washington Medical Center in Seattle, WA. After completing his residency training, Dr. Long completed an Endourological Society Fellowship in robotics, laparoscopy, and endo-urology at the University of Washington. He is a member of the American Urological Association, American Board of Urology, American Association of Clinical Urologist, Society of Endourology, and Society of laparoscopic Surgeons. He is currently the director of urological robotic surgery and the chief of the robotics section at Good Samaritan Regional Medical Center. Dr. Long serves as a robotic surgery proctor for Intuitive Surgical and an asst clinical professor of Surgery and serves a board member of Waveform Lithotripsy.

Contents

Preface

It is a distinct pleasure to serve as an editor for this book dedicated to nephrolithiasis, laser fragmentation, and a novel use of a well-known surgical technology.

Nephrolithiasis or nephrocalcinosis (the formation of kidney stones or renal calculi) is a common problem worldwide with substantial consequences in terms of morbidities and economic burden. The incidence of kidney stones has increased in recent decades along with a significant narrowing of the gender gap. Similarly, the incidence of kidney stone formation in the pediatric population is on a gradual incline.

In this text, we present a host of international scientists/authors who have composed and contributed updates and some advances to the existing body of literature as it relates to the pathophysiology of stone formation; laser pulse–induced calculus damage; the increased incidence and recurrence of kidney stones in the pediatric population; a comprehensive review of inheritance patterns; diagnosis, medical treatment, and prevention of cystinuria; and finally recent trends in the novel utility of extracorporeal shock wave lithotripsy, as commonly used modality of treatment for kidney stones.

The first chapter of Section 1 is dedicated to discussing our current understanding of the pathophysiology of nephrocalcinosis. In a comprehensive manner, the authors explore and review the genetics of predisposing conditions to nephrocalcinosis. This chapter explores and compares the mechanisms that propagate renal and vascular calcifications, including tubular calcinosis and interstitial calcinoses. Furthermore, it touches on the molecular factors that contribute to cell-driven calcification such as phosphates, oxidative stress, hormones, and microRNAs.

In the subsequent chapter, the authors underscore the high rate of recurrent kidney stones in the pediatric population and the importance of metaphylaxis, including how a thorough assessment and planning are essential to provide accurate and effective therapy. When considering dietary modifications, a risk and benefit assessment is particularly important in this population since their development is an ongoing process. If dietary modification is not sufficient, medical treatment must be implemented.

The final chapter of Section 1 provides a very detailed review of the rare genetic condition of cystinuria. At present, preventative medical treatment is the mainstay of treatment aimed at reducing the calculi burden to avoid the risk of chronic renal impairment. Our evolving understanding of the genetic mutations implicated in this will eventually foster targeted treatments.

In a section devoted to modalities of treatment, we include a chapter on the physics of laser fragmentation of calculi. While laser lithotripsy is now a preferred treatment option for urolithiasis, the mechanism of laser pulse–induced calculus damage is still not fully understood. They use a combination of a high-speed camera with hydrophone, pendulum, and Schlieren imaging methods to characterize cavitation bubble, shock wave, and fiber burn-back and retropulsion. This is particularly important as replacement of damaged fibers and retreatment rates accrue a significant healthcare expense.

The final chapter covers novel uses of extracorporeal shockwave lithotripsy (ESWL). Since its introduction in the 1980s, ESWL has been offered as a minimally invasive method of treating renal calculi. In recent years, ESWL has been used successfully in the management of various other anatomical sites.

In recent decades, we have enhanced our understanding of the pathophysiology and genetics of rare and common causes of kidney stones. With our evolving understanding of the epidemiology, biology, and genetics of nephrolithiasis and the advances in therapeutic technologies, we have made significant progress in patient care. Furthermore, advances in the medical management and surgical technologies have allowed us to embellish the optimal outcomes in the management of complex kidney stone disease.

This body of work, and the ongoing investigations to follow, will continue to strengthen our understanding of nephrolithiasis and help us to get closer to developing sophisticated tool to offer even more definitive treatment options for patients.

Dr. Layron Long
Samaritan Urology
Chief of Robotic Section
Director of Urological Robotic Surgery
Fellowship trained in Robotic, Laparoscopy and Endourology
Good Samaritan Regional Medical Center
Corvallis, OR, USA

Section 1

Pathophysiology of Nephrolithiasis

Chapter 1

Understanding the Pathophysiology of Nephrocalcinosis

Giovanna Priante, Monica Ceol, Liliana Terrin,
Lisa Gianesello, Federica Quaggio,
Dorella Del Prete and Franca Anglani

Additional information is available at the end of the chapter

http://dx.doi.org/10.5772/intechopen.69895

Abstract

Many *in vitro* and *in vivo* studies on the mechanisms underlying calcium nephrolithiasis have provided evidence of a frequently associated condition, i.e., a microscopic renal crystal deposition that can occur within the tubular lumen (intratubular nephrocalcinosis) or in the interstitium (interstitial nephrocalcinosis). Medullary nephrocalcinosis is the typical pattern seen in 98% of cases of human nephrocalcinosis, with calcification clustering around each renal pyramid. It is common in patients with metabolic conditions that predispose them to renal calcium stones. Cortical nephrocalcinosis is rare and usually results from severe destructive disease of the cortex. It has been described in chronic glomerulonephritis, but often in association with another factor, such as an increased calcium ingestion, acute cortical necrosis, chronic pyelonephritis or trauma. The most accredited hypothesis to explain the onset of interstitial nephrocalcinosis is purely physicochemical, relating to spontaneous Ca_2PO_4 crystallization in the interstitium due to oversaturation of Ca_2PO_4salts in this milieu. The theory that nephrocalcinosis is a process driven by osteogenic cells was first proposed by our group. We review nephrocalcinosis in terms of its definition, genetic associations, and putative mechanisms, pointing out how much evidence in the literature suggests that it may have some features in common with, and pathogenic links to vascular calcification.

Keywords: nephrocalcinosis, genetics, Randall's plaque, calcium crystals, vascular calcification, osteogenic transdifferentiation

1. Introduction

Nephrolithiasis is a common disease, typically occurring between 30 and 60 years of age. It is the most often-diagnosed chronic condition involving the kidney, after hypertension. The symptoms and consequences are not life threatening for the majority of patients, but stones in the urinary tract are a major cause of morbidity, hospitalization, and days lost from work [1]. The incidence of nephrolithiasis is increasing. In Italy, for example, the number of patients given hospital treatment for this condition rose between 1988 and 1993 from 60,000 to 80,000 a year. About 12,000 patients a year required surgical treatment or urological maneuvers, and the number of extracorporeal shock wave lithotripsy sessions administered amounted to approximately 50,000 a year [2].

The metabolic characteristics of the urinary stones identified in patients with nephrolithiasis vary, but the most common (accounting for 75% of all cases) are calcium-containing stones. Calcium oxalate (CaOx) is the primary component of most stones [3], often combined with some calcium phosphate (CaP), which may form the stone's initial nidus. Crystal retention in the kidney is essential to stone formation and this occurs with several different patterns of deposition in the kidneys of stone formers, each pattern being associated with specific types of stone. Patients with idiopathic CaOx stones have white deposits on their papillae called "Randall's plaque" [4]. Biopsies of these areas reveal interstitial deposits of CaP in the form of biological apatite, which first develop in the basement membrane of the thin loops of Henle and which contain layers of protein matrix. These deposits may extend down to the tip of the papilla and, if the overlying urothelium is denuded, the exposed plaque can become an attachment site for stones [5]. Stones seem to start as deposits of amorphous CaP overlying the exposed plaque, interspersed with urinary proteins. With time, more layers of protein and mineral are deposited, and the mineral phase becomes predominantly CaOx.

By contrast, in patients whose stones consist mainly of CaP (apatite or brushite), these stones are not attached to plaque. Instead, many collecting ducts fill with crystal deposits that occupy the tubule lumen and may protrude from the openings in the ducts of Bellini. Generally speaking, most stone formers studied to date have had crystal deposits in the medullary collecting ducts, with the exception of those with idiopathic CaOx stones, who have no intratubular deposits, but abundant deposits of apatite in the papillary interstitium.

Calcium nephrolithiasis, the most common renal form of stone disease, is defined as the formation of macroscopic concretions of inorganic and organic material in the renal calyces and/or pelvis. Many *in vitro* and *in vivo* studies on the mechanisms underlying calcium nephrolithiasis have produced evidence of this condition frequently being associated with nephrocalcinosis, a condition involving microscopic renal crystal deposition.

2. Nephrocalcinosis

Strictly speaking, the term "nephrocalcinosis" refers to the generalized deposition of CaP or CaOX in the kidney, which can occur within the tubular lumen (*intratubular nephrocalcinosis*) or in the interstitium (*interstitial nephrocalcinosis*). Some authorities restrict the definition of nephrocalcinosis to the deposition of CaP crystals in the interstitium. Randall's plaque could be an example of interstitial nephrocalcinosis.

It has been suggested in Refs. [6, 7] that nephrocalcinosis should be divided into three categories: *molecular nephrocalcinosis*, involving an increase in renal intracellular calcium without any crystal formation and essentially reflecting the renal dysfunction of hypercalcemia; *microscopic nephrocalcinosis*, in which CaP or CaOX crystals are visible on light microscopy, but not radiologically; and macroscopic nephrocalcinosis, when calcification is visible radiologically or on ultrasound scans. Nephrocalcinosis does not necessarily lead to renal stones, and renal stones may occur without any apparent macroscopic nephrocalcinosis, so these two conditions are distinct but closely related [6].

As for the sites involved, nephrocalcinosis can be divided into cortical and medullary nephrocalcinosis.

Cortical nephrocalcinosis is rare and usually results from severe destructive disease of the cortex. This condition has been described in chronic glomerulonephritis, though often in association with another factor, such as an increased calcium ingestion, acute cortical necrosis, chronic pyelonephritis, or trauma [8, 9], autosomal recessive polycystic kidney disease, primary and secondary oxalosis, chronic renal allograft rejection, or benign nodular cortical nephrocalcinosis [7]. Three different patterns of cortical nephrocalcinosis have been identified radiologically [10]. In the most common pattern, there is a thin peripheral band of calcification, often extending into the septal cortex. In a second type, there is a double line of calcification along the two sides of the necrotic zone in the cortex (what Lloyd Thomas et al. called "tram line" calcification in describing the pattern of nephrocalcinosis seen in obstetric cases of cortical necrosis [11]). The least common pattern consists of multiple punctate calcifications randomly distributed in the renal cortex.

Medullary nephrocalcinosis is the typical form seen in 98% of cases of human nephrocalcinosis. It forms clusters of calcification around each renal pyramid. It is common in patients with metabolic conditions (several of which are monogenic diseases) that predispose them to renal calcium stones. Knowing which genes are involved can help to shed light on the mechanisms behind nephrocalcinosis.

2.1. Genetics of Conditions predisposing to medullary nephrocalcinosis

Stone initiation and growth is prompted by the urine becoming supersaturated with a solute of calcium, oxalate, uric acid, and cystine, which leads the dissolved salts to condense into solids, thus forming the stone. But urinary CaOx supersaturation is a common finding in normal individuals too, who develop no stones. This is most likely due to the presence of crystallization inhibitors such as citrate or pyrophosphate in their urine. In addition to the concentration of solutes, urinary pH is a crucially important factor influencing crystal solubility. Supersaturation and crystallization in the urine also rely on the presence of macromolecules capable of binding and forming complexes with Ca and Ox. Mammalian urine contains numerous macromolecules that inhibit crystal formation, growth, and aggregation in the kidney. Levels of supersaturation and crystallization are kept under control by the proper functioning of a variety of cells lining the renal tubules [12, 13].

Conditions predisposing to medullary nephrocalcinosis may be either those that raise the urinary concentration of inductors of calcium crystal deposition or those that lower the concentration of the inhibitors of this process. The former category includes hypercalciuria, hyperoxaluria, the latter hypocitraturia and hypomagnesuria. Renal tubular acidosis (RTA), on the other hand, is responsible for changes in urinary pH, which has a fundamental role in favoring crystallization. In some cases, there may also be specific anatomical abnormalities that predispose to the onset of nephrocalcinosis, as in medullary sponge kidney (MSK).

Several genetic disorders have been found associated with conditions that predispose individuals to the development and progression of nephrocalcinosis. Most of them are tubular disorders associated with epithelial cellular and paracellular ion transport disruptions that result in the urinary excretion of higher levels of calcium, phosphate or oxalate and lower levels of citrate and magnesium. **Table 1** shows the genetic basis for the link between some inherited disorders and medullary nephrocalcinosis [7]. **Figure 1** shows the list of intrarenal transport defects that prompt a dysfunctional renal handling of the two most important divalent cations Ca^{2+} and Mg^{2+} [14]. As can be noted, not all cation-handling disorders are associated with nephrocalcinosis.

The kidney handles calcium, phosphate, and oxalate in the proximal tubules, in the thick ascending limb (TAL) of the loop of Henle, and in the distal convolute tubule (DCT), shown in **Figure 2** [6]. Knowing the site where the tubular exchanger and transporter proteins involved in regulating urinary calcium, phosphate, and oxalate work help us better understand the mechanisms underlying nephrocalcinosis.

Bearing in mind that 98% of interstitial crystal deposition occurs in the medulla around each pyramid, Sayer et al. proposed the model of nephrocalcinosis shown in **Figure 3**.

We focus our attention on the genetic defects that alter the kidney's homeostatic capacity.

2.2. Renal calcium handling

Of all the calcium filtered by the kidney, 98% is reabsorbed by the tubules, with the proximal tubule reabsorbing about 65%, the TAL of the loop of Henle accounting for approximately 20–25%, and 8–10% being reabsorbed in the distal tubule [15]. Hypercalciuria is an important, identifiable, and reversible nephrocalcinosis risk factor. It is a complex trait, caused by both environmental and genetic factors. It is not a disease per se, but represents the upper end of a continuum, rather like height, weight, and blood pressure, and—like these polygenic traits—urinary calcium excretion should be considered a graded risk factor [16]. **Table 2** shows a summary of the clinically and experimentally identified monogenic causes of hypercalciuria, pointing to the genetic causes of renal calcium leak.

It is worth remembering that the crystallization of calcium salts is a physiological event linked to biomineralization, i.e., the capacity of calcium, like other inorganic crystalline or non-crystalline minerals, to interact with and deposit around biomolecules, becoming an integral part of organic tissues to provide hardness and strength. Biomineralization is often arbitrarily distinguished as physiological or pathological. It would be more appropriate to say that pathological calcium crystallization is a physiological process occurring in the wrong place and at the wrong time [17]. Nephrocalcinosis might fit this definition.

http://dx.doi.org/10.5772/intechopen.69895

Gene	Protein	Disorder	Mode of inheritance
ATP6V1B1	β1 Subunit of H^+ - ATPase	Distal renal tubular acidosis (dRTA)	AR
ATPV0A4	α4 Subunit of H^+- ATPase	Distal renal tubular acidosis (dRTA) with neural deafness at birth or late onset	AR
SLC12A1	Sodium-potassium-chloride transporter (NKCC2)	Bartter syndrome type 1	AR
KCNJ1	Potassium channel (ROMK1)	Bartter syndrome type 2	AR
BSND	Barttin	Bartter syndrome type 4	AR
CLCNKB	Chloride channel ClC-Kb	Bartter syndrome type 3	AR
CASR	Calcium-sensing receptor (CasR)	Hypocalcemia with hypercalciuria	AD
CFTR	ATP-binding cassette transporter	Cystic fibrosis	
CLDN16	Claudin-16, tight junction	Familial hypomagnesemia with hypercalciuria and nephrocalcinosis	AR
CLDN19	Claudin-19, tight junction	Familial hypomagnesemia with hypercalciuria and nephrocalcinosis with ocular impairment	AR
SLC4A1	AE1	Distal renal tubular acidosis (dRTA) with neural deafness at birth or late inset	AD
SLC34A3	Sodium-dependent phosphate transporter protein 2C (NPT2C)	Hereditary hypophosphatemic rickets with hypercalciuria (HHRH)	AR
CLCN5	Chloride channel 5 (ClC-5)	Dent disease 1	XLR
OCRL	Phosphatidylinositol 4,5-bisphosphate 5-phosphatase (OCRL1)	Dent disease 2 or Lowe's syndrome	XLR
PHEX	Phosphate-regulating endopeptidase	Hypophosphatemic rickets	XLD
FAM20A	Pseudokinase FAM20A	MacGibbon-Lubinsky sindrome	AD
AGXT	Alanine glyoxylate aminotransferase	Primary hyperoxaluria (PH type I)	AR
GRHPR	Glyoxylate reductase	Primary hyperoxaluria (PH type 2)	AR
ELN, LIMK1	Elastin	Williams-Beuren syndrome (WBS)	AR

Gene	Protein	Disorder	Mode of inheritance
GDNF	Glial cell line-derived neurotrophic factor	Medullary sponge kidney (MSK)	AD
SLC7A9	B(0,+)-type amino acid Transporter 1 (BAT1)	Cystinuria	AD
ADCY10	Adenylate Cyclase 10, Soluble	Familial idiopathic hypercalciuria	AD
SCNN1G/B	Renal epithelium channel (βENaC and αENaC)	Liddle syndrome	AD
ATP7B	Copper-transporting ATP-ase	Wilson syndrome	AR

AD, autosomal dominant; AR, autosomal recessive; XLR, X-linked recessive; XLD, X-linked dominant.

Table 1. Inherited disorders associated to medullary nephrocalcinosis (NC).

2.3. Renal phosphate handling

The kidney's control over systemic phosphate homeostasis is crucial. About 80% of filtered phosphate is reabsorbed from the urine by transporters located in the proximal tubule and mostly in the juxtamedullary nephrons (**Figure 2**). At least three transporters are responsible for renal phosphate reabsorption, and they are precisely regulated by various cellular mechanisms and factors [18]. They are members of the Type II NA^+-dependent phosphate cotransporter family encoded by the SLC34A1, SLC34A3, and SLC20A2 genes. Though it is not a

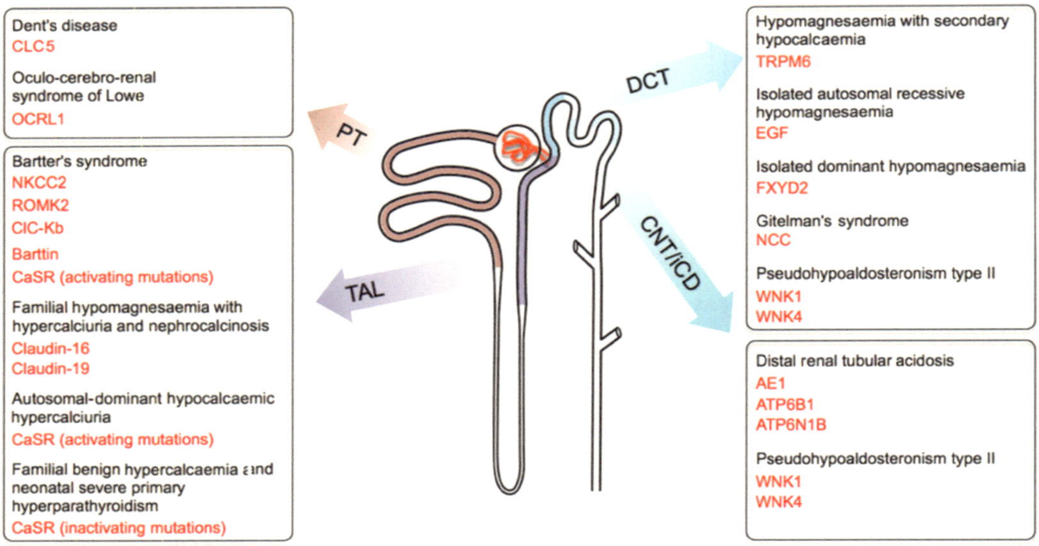

Figure 1. Schematic representation of the nephron listing the predominant origins of intrarenal transport defects causing dysfunctional renal handling of divalent cations. This figure was originally published in Ref. [14].

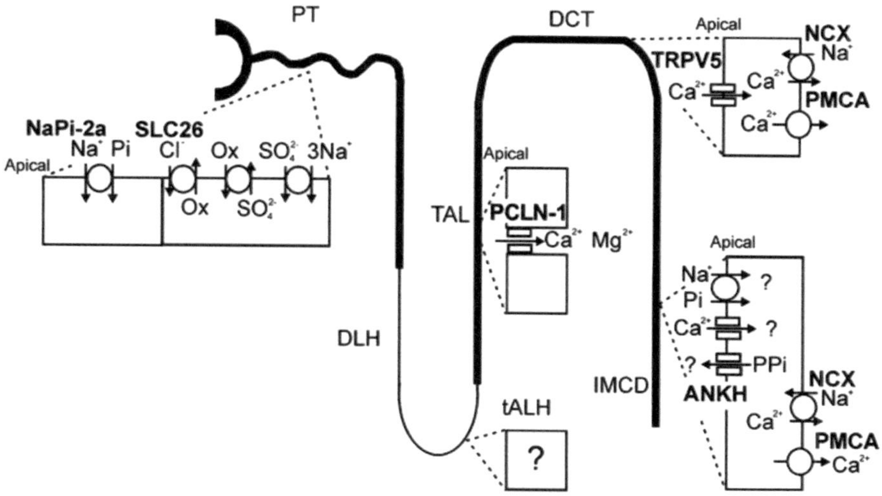

Figure 2. Tubular transport of calcium, phosphate, and oxalate. A nephron map of exchanger and transporter proteins involved in the regulation of urinary calcium, phosphate and oxalate is shown. In the proximal tubule (PT) apical Na/Pi cotransporters (NaPi-2a) mediate phosphate reabsorption, whereas several anion exchange proteins (including those of the SLC26 family) mediate transcellular oxalate (Ox) secretion and recycling. There is no evidence for calcium or phosphate transport in the thin descending limb (DLH) or the thin ascending limb (tALH)of the loop of Henle. The TAL of Henle allows paracellular calcium (and magnesium) reabsorption via paracellin channels (PCLN-1). The distal convoluted tubule (DCT) allows for regulated transcellular reabsorption of calcium via apical TRPV5 and the basolateral NCX, together with the basolateral PMCA. A calcium entry pathway exists within the IMCD, the molecular identity of which remains uncertain. It is likely that Na/Pi isoforms are also present in this nephron segment and their physiological function may be linked to the PPi transporter protein ANKH. Basolateral calcium exporters NCX and PMCA are also present in the collecting duct. This figure was originally published in Ref. [6].

transporter protein, the Na+/H+ exchanger regulatory factor (NHERF1) plays a crucial part in renal phosphate transport by binding to SLC34A1 in the proximal tubule. Alterations in the genes encoding these transporters result in phosphate wasting, and consequent hyperphosphaturia (**Table 3**). For the sake of completeness, **Table 3** also includes renal phosphate handling impairments due to extrarenal inherited defects.

2.4. Renal oxalate handling

Urinary oxalate is the most important risk factor for CaOx nephrocalcinosis/nephrolithiasis. Oxalate is filtered freely at the glomerulus [6]. Anion exchange proteins in the proximal tubule mediate oxalate excretion and recycling at the brush border membrane (**Figure 2**). These proteins belong to the SLC26 family, and they allow oxalate loss in exchange for chloride, then uptake oxalate in exchange for sulfate loss, energized by Na-sulfate transport in the proximal tubules [19]. The main causes of hyperoxaluria relate, however, to genetic defects that alter glyoxylate metabolism in the liver and erythrocytes, leading to endogenous oxalate overproduction. These hereditary autosomal recessive forms of hyperoxaluria are called primary hyperoxaluria type I, type II, and type III [20]. Defects in the genes responsible for oxalate reabsorption have recently been reported too. Recessive mutations in SLC26A1 gene were identified in two unrelated individuals with calcium oxalate kidney stones. Functional experiments have

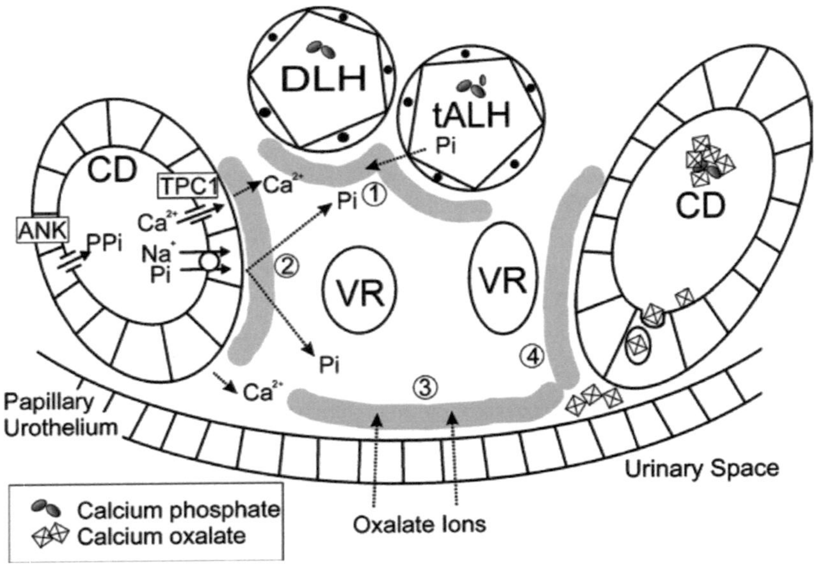

Figure 3. Renal papillary model of nephrocalcinosis. Collecting ducts (CD) together with descending loops of Henle (DLH) and ascending thin loops of Henle (tALH) and vasa recta (VR) are shown through a cross-section of a renal papilla. Possible initial sites of nephrocalcinosis are shown as shaded regions. Mechanisms leading to calcification may include: (1) Pi permeability at the papillary thin loops of Henle would allow interstitial loading of phosphate; (2) collecting duct absorption of calcium, possibly via apical calcium channels (e.g., TPC1) and basolateral calcium exit would allow delivery of calcium ions to the interstitium; Na/Pi cotransport at a collecting duct location would also provide additional phosphate ions, which may be derived from PPi delivery into the lumen via ANK; (3) concentration of oxalate from the urinary space into the papillary interstitium allows delivery of oxalate ions; (4) intraluminal crystal formation, both from the loop of Henle (calcium phosphate) and collecting duct (calcium oxalate) may adhere to collecting duct epithelial surfaces, then by endocytosis/transcytosis the crystals are delivered to the papillary interstitium and accumulate. Dissolution by epithelial cells or by interstitial cells (including macrophages) may provide a clearance mechanism. This figure was originally published in Ref. [6].

shown that these mutations resulted in decreased transporter activity [21], thus confirming their role in the disease. In the SLC26A6 gene has also recently been described a single nucleotide polymorphism associated with increased calcium oxalate kidney stones [22]. **Table 4** summarizes what we know about the genetics of hyperoxaluria.

2.5. Renal citrate handling

Citrate is filtrated freely at the glomerulus. In humans, from 65 to 90% of the filtered citrate is reabsorbed, mainly in the proximal tubule [23]. Urinary citrate is an important calcium chelator, consequently reducing the potential of calcium and oxalate to interact. In addition, citrate binds crystals' surface preventing their adhesion to renal epithelial cells [24]. It is intriguing that oxalate transport by SLC26A6 and citrate transport by the sodium dicarboxyl cotransporter SLC13A2—both located in the apical membrane of the proximal tubules and small intestine—have been found to interact. This was demonstrated in SLC26A6 KO mice, which are not only hyperoxaluric, but also hypocitraturic [25]. Hypocitraturia is a known risk factor for the development

Gene	Protein	Disorder	Mode of inheritance
ATP6V1B1	β1 Subunit of H^+ - ATPase	Distal renal tubular acidosis (dRTA)	AD
ATPV0A4	α4 Subunit of H^+ - ATPase	Distal renal tubular acidosis (dRTA) with neural deafness at birth or late onset	AR
SLC12A1	Sodium-potassium-chloride transporter (NKCC2)	Bartter syndrome type 1	AR
KCNJ1	Potassium channel (ROMK1)	Bartter syndrome type 2	AD
CLCNKB	Chloride channel ClC-Kb	Bartter syndrome type 3	AR
BSND	Barttin	Bartter syndrome type 4	AR
MAGED2	Melanoma associated antigen D2	Bartter syndrome type 5	XLR
CASR	Calcium-sensing receptor (CasR)	Hypercalciuria with hypocalcemia	AD
G6PC	Glucose-6-phosphatase	Glycogen storage disease type 1a	AR
FAH	Fumarylacetoacetase	Tyrosinemia type 1	AR
ATP7B	Copper-transporting ATP-ase	Wilson disease	AR
CLCN5	Chloride channel 5 (ClC-5)	Dent disease 1	XLR
OCRL	Phosphatidylinositol 4,5-bisphosphate 5-phosphatase (OCRL1)	Dent disease 2, Lowe syndrome	XLR
CLDN16	Claudin-16, tight junction	Familial hypomagnesemia with hypercalciuria	AR
CLDN19	Claudin-19, tight junction	Familial hypomagnesemia with hypercalciuria	AR
SLC34A1	Sodium-phosphate transport protein 2A	Fanconi renal tubular syndrome 2	AR
ADCY10	Adenylate Cyclase 10, Soluble	Familial idiopathic hypercalciuria	AD
KLOTHO	Regulator of calcium homeostasis (Klotho)	Tumoral calcinosis, hyperphosphatemic	AR

AD, autosomal dominant; AR, autosomal recessive; XLR, X-linked recessive.

Table 2. Monogenic forms of hypercalciuria: kidney as the primary defect.

Gene	Protein	Disorder	Mode of inheritance
SLC34A1	Sodium-phosphate transport protein 2A	Fanconi renal tubular syndrome 2, Hypophosphatemic nephrolithiasis/ osteoporosis-1	AD
SLC34A3	Sodium-phosphate transport protein 2C	Hereditary hypophosphatemic rickets with hypercalciuria (HHRH)	AR
SLC9A3R1	Na^+/H^+ exchange regulatory cofactor NHE-RF1	Hypophosphatemic nephrolithiasis/ osteoporosis-2	AD
FGF23	Fibroblast growth factor 23	Hypophosphatemic ricket	AD
KLOTHO	Regulator of calcium homeostasis (Klotho)	Tumoral calcinosis, hyperphosphatemic	AR
GALNT3	Polypeptide N-acetylgalactosaminyltransferase 3	Tumoral calcinosis, hyperphosphatemic	AR
PHEX	Phosphate-regulating neutral endopeptidase	Hypophosphatemic rickets	XLD
FAM20C	Extracellular serine/threonine protein kinase	Raine syndrome	AR
FGFR1	Fibroblast growth factor receptor 1	Osteoglophonic dysplasia	AD
DMP1	Dentin matrix acidic phosphoprotein 1	Hypophosphatemic rickets	AR

AD, autosomal dominant; AR, autosomal recessive; XLD, X-linked dominant.

Table 3. Genetic basis of altered renal phosphate handling.

of nephrocalcinosis/nephrolithiasis. No monogenic form of hypocitraturia has been reported so far, whereas genetic associations have been demonstrated between polymorphisms in the VDR and SLC13A2 genes and hypocitraturia [26, 27]. Very recently, Rendina et al. [28] provided evidence of an epistatic interaction between VDR and SLC13A2 in the pathogenesis of hypocitraturia. This may come as no surprise because the active form of vitamin D in the nephron uses VDR to modulate citrate metabolism and transport [26]. Finally, Shah et al. [29] have suggested

Disorder	Gene	Protein	Mode of inheritance
Hyperoxaluria type I	AGXT	Serine-pyruvate aminotransferase	AR
Hyperoxaluria type II	GRHPR	Glyoxylate reductase/ hydroxypyruvate reductase	AR
Hyperoxaluria type III	HOGA1	4-hydroxy-2-oxoglutarate aldolase, mitochondria	AR
Calcium oxalate kidney stones	SLC26A1	Sulfate anion transporter 1	AR

PH, primary hyperoxaluria; AR, autosomal recessive.

Table 4. Inherited disorders of renal oxalate handling.

other genetic influences on citrate handling too: they propose a codominant inheritance of alleles at a single locus based on their trimodal frequency distribution of citrate excretion.

2.6. Renal magnesium handling

Hypomagnesuria is the biochemical abnormality found in about 19% of kidney stone patients, alone or in association with other biochemical abnormalities [30]. The kidney has a key role in maintaining a normal magnesium balance. The TAL of the loop of Henle and the DCT are crucially important in regulating serum magnesium levels and body magnesium content (**Figure 2**). Understanding the molecular defects behind rare genetic magnesium loss disorders has greatly contributed to our understanding of renal magnesium handling. About 80% of all plasma magnesium is filtered through the glomeruli, and 15–20% of it is reabsorbed by the proximal tubules, and 55–70% by the cortical TAL [31]. Magnesium is reabsorbed via a paracellular pathway in this nephron segment. Members of the claudin family of tight junction proteins have been attributed a role in controlling magnesium and calcium permeability of the paracellular pathway (**Figure 4**) [31]. Although only 5–10% of the filtered magnesium is reabsorbed in the DCT, this process is finely regulated and plays an important part in determining its final urinary excretion [31, 32].

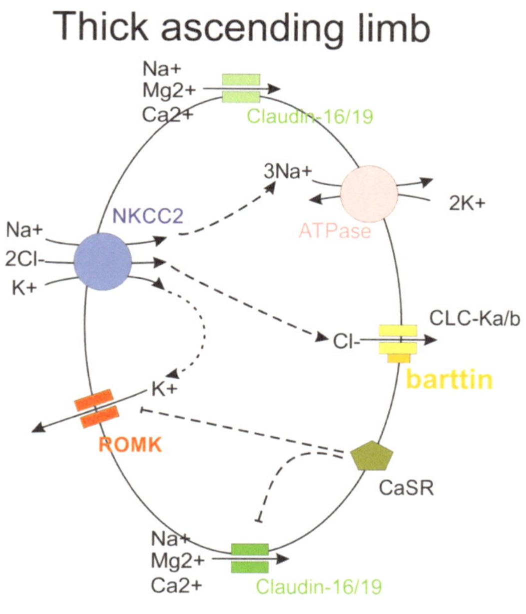

Figure 4. Magnesium reabsorption in the cortical thick ascending limb (TAL) of Henle's loop and in the distal convoluted tubule (DCT). The key proteins influencing magnesium reabsorption are indicated. Magnesium reabsorption in the TAL is passive and occurs through the paracellular pathway. The driving force is the lumen-positive transcellular voltage, which is generated by the transcellular reabsorption of NaCl and the potassium recycling back to the tubular fluid via ROMK. Magnesium transport through DCT cells is active and depends on the negative membrane plasma potential. This mechanism seems to depend on a sodium gradient that results from the coordinate action of NCCT, Na-K-ATPase and Kir4.1.

Gene	Protein	Disorder	Mode of inheritance
SLC12A1	Sodium-potassium-chloride transporter (NKCC2)	Bartter syndrome type 1	AR
KCNJ1	Potassium channel (ROMK1)	Bartter syndrome type 2	AR
CLCNKB	Chloride channel ClC-Kb	Bartter syndrome type 3	AR
BSND	Barttin	Bartter syndrome type 4	AR
CLDN16	Claudin-16, tight junction	Familial hypomagnesemia with hypercalciuria and nephrocalcinosis	AR
CLDN19	Claudin-19, tight junction	Familial hypomagnesemia with hypercalciuria and nephrocalcinosis with ocular impairment	AR
CASR	Calcium-sensing receptor (CasR)	Hypercalciuric hypercalcemia	AD
FXYD2	Gamma subunit Na/K/ATPase	Hypomagnesemia 2, renal	AD
TRPM6	TRPM6 cation channel	Hypomagnesemia 1, intestinal with secondary hypocalcemia	AR
SLC12A3	NaCl cotrasporter (NCCT)	Gitelman syndrome	AR
EGF	Epidermal growth factor (Pro-EGF)	Hypomagnesemia 4, renal	AR
KCNA1	Kv1.1 Potassium channel	Myokymia 1 with hypomagnesemia	AD
KCNJ10	Kir4.1 potassium channel	SESAME syndrome	AR
HNF1B	HNF1β transcription factor	HNF1B nephropathy	AD

Note: AD = autosomal dominant; AR = autosomal recessive.

Table 5. Inherited disorders of renal magnesium loss.

Hereditary forms of hypomagnesemia include rare, genetically determined disorders that may affect renal magnesium handling either primarily or secondarily. **Table 5** summarizes the spectrum of underlying genetic defects [31].

2.7. Pyrophosphaturia

Pyrophosphate (PPi) is present in urine and can contribute 50% CaOx monohydrate (COM) crystal growth inhibition in the collecting duct and up to 80% in the urine [33, 34]. It has been postulated that hypopyrophosphaturia is a metabolic risk factor for recurrent stone formers [35]. That the concentration of inorganic PPi is higher in urine than in plasma cannot fully explain the origin of urinary PPi, but does suggest that it is somehow either secreted into the tubule or generated locally [36]. PPi is generated mostly in the mitochondria, and it is a byproduct of about 190 biochemical reactions. The PPi end product must be promptly removed to ensure irreversible, one-way reactions. PPi may be removed in three ways: by hydrolysis via cytoplasmic phosphatases; by PPi compartmentalization; or by its exportation from the cytoplasm via a transporter such as ANKH protein, which is located in the principal cells of the renal collecting duct (**Figure 2**) [6, 37]. Many authors now assume that PPi is removed from the cell by this third means, although the exact physiological function of the ANKH protein has never been clarified [36]. Underexpression or loss of activity of ANK (the mouse homolog of ANKH) is believed to lead to CaP deposition in numerous tissues, due to loss of PPi's inhibitory effects on CaP formation, and to the ubiquitous nature of CaP mineralization [38]. The majority of known ANKH mutations are assumed to be of the gain-of-function type, however, and are responsible for clinical phenotypes characterized by calcium PPi deposition in the joints, i.e., calcium pyrophosphate deposition disease [39]. Loss-of-function mutations presumably responsible for the loss of ANKH activity and a lower extracellular PPi were detected in patients with craniometaphyseal dysplasia, which is characterized by overgrowth and sclerosis of the facial bones and abnormal long bone modeling. No renal calcification was seen in association with this disease, however. Unlike bone, ion content in the tubular environment varies considerably, and the picture is further complicated by various reabsorption mechanisms, which may in turn be affected by a negative feedback from the tubular ion content [36]. This might explain why ANKH loss of function does not cause nephrocalcinosis or kidney stones.

2.8. Regulation of urinary acidification

One of the main functions of the kidney is to keep the systemic acid-base chemistry constant. The kidney has evolved so that it can regulate blood acidity by means of three key functions: (1) by reabsorbing the $HCO3^-$ filtered through the glomeruli to prevent its excretion in the urine; (2) by generating a sufficient quantity of new $HCO3^-$ to compensate for the loss of $HCO3^-$ due to dietary metabolic H+ loads and loss of $HCO3^-$ in the urea cycle; and (3) by excreting $HCO3^-$ (or metabolizable organic anions) following a systemic base load [40]. For the kidney to be able to perform these functions, various types of cell throughout the nephron have to respond to changes in acid-base chemistry by modulating specific ion transport and/or metabolic processes in a coordinated fashion, such that the urine and renal vein chemistry is adjusted appropriately. The kidney contributes to acid-base homeostasis by recovering filtered bicarbonate in the proximal tubule. Distally, intercalated cells of the collecting duct generate new bicarbonate, which is consumed by the titration of non-volatile acid [41].

The renal tubular acidosis (RTA) syndromes encompass a disparate group of tubular transport defects that share the inability to secrete hydrogen ions (H^+). This inability results in failure to excrete acid in the form of ammonium ($NH4^+$) ions and titratable acids or to reabsorb some of the filtered bicarbonate ($HCO3^-$). Either situation coincides with a drop in plasma bicarbonate levels, leading to chronic metabolic acidosis. Much of the morbidity of RTA syndromes is attributable to the systemic consequences of chronic metabolic acidosis, including growth retardation, bone disease, and kidney stones [42].

Dysfunction of the proximal tubules, where approximately 90% of the bicarbonate is reabsorbed, leads to proximal RTA [43], whereas malfunctioning of the intercalated cells in the collecting ducts accounts for all known genetic causes of distal RTA (dRTA).

Inherited proximal RTA is a rare disorder that may be inherited as an autosomal recessive or dominant trait [44]. The more common autosomal recessive form has been associated with mutations in the basolateral sodium bicarbonate cotransporter NBCe1, encoded by the SLC4A4 gene. Mutations in this transporter lead to a reduced activity and/or trafficking, thus, disrupting the normal bicarbonate reabsorption process in the proximal tubules [45]. As an isolated defect of bicarbonate transport, proximal RTA is rare. It is more often associated with Fanconi syndrome, which features urinary wastage of solutes such as phosphate, uric acid, glucose, amino acids, and low-molecular-weight proteins, as well as bicarbonate. The distal acidification mechanisms remain intact, however, and acid urine can still be produced. The clinical phenotype is of a metabolic acidosis with hypokalemia; metabolic bone disease is common, but nephrocalcinosis and nephrolithiasis are rare [46].

In contrast, 80% of cases of distal RTA (dRTA) are associated with medullary nephrocalcinosis. The molecular basis underlying primary dRTA is a defective functioning of alpha intercalated cells [41]. The molecular defects behind proximal and distal RTA are listed in **Table 6**.

The clinical signs and symptoms of dRTA can vary, depending on the underlying mutation: patients may reveal a mild metabolic acidosis after the incidental detection of kidney stones, or they may have severe health issues with failure to thrive and growth retardation in children, rickets, severe metabolic acidosis, and nephrocalcinosis. Kidney stones in dRTA consist of CaP due to the release of Ca and Pi from bone to buffer the acidosis, leading to hypercalciuria and consequent CaP precipitation due to an alkaline pH [47].

2.9. Macromoleculuria

The formation of crystal aggregates involves interaction between crystals and urinary macromolecules (UMs) that serve as an adhesive. The number of UMs isolated in urine has been

Disorder	Gene	Protein	Mode of inheritance
Distal RTA type1	SLC4A1	AE1	AR
	SLC4A1	AE1	AD
	ATP6V1B1	β1 Subunit of H^+ - ATPase	AR with early onset hearing loss
	ATPV0A4	α4 Subunit of H^+- ATPase	AR with later onset hearing loss
Proximal RTA type2	SLC4A4	Sodium bicarbonate cotransporter 1 (NBC1)	AR
Combined Proximal and Distal RTA type3	Ca2	Carbonic anhydrase 2 (CAH2)	AR

PH, primary hyperoxaluria; AR, autosomal recessive.

Table 6. The inherited renal tubular acidoses.

steadily increasing, and they now form a large group of proteins and some glycosaminoglycans [48, 49]. The main macromolecules involved in crystallization are summarized in **Table 7**.

Although the role of these proteins in stone formation is still far from clear, coating of the crystals by the urinary macromolecules seems to prevent crystal aggregation or at least delay it for long enough for the urine to transit through the kidney.

An inhibitory role has repeatedly been confirmed for osteopontin (OPN) [50–54], which is synthesized in the kidney and excreted in the urine in concentrations that suffice to inhibit CaOx crystallization. No naturally occurring mutations in the SSP1 gene encoding OPN have ever been reported in human diseases, but SSP1 polymorphisms have been associated with the risk of nephrolithiasis [55–57].

Tamm-Horsfall protein (THP), also called uromodulin, is a kidney-specific protein synthesized by cells in the TAL of the loop of Henle. It is the most abundant protein in human urine. It is a potent inhibitor of crystal aggregation *in vitro*, and its ablation *in vivo* predisposes one of the two existing mouse models to spontaneous intrarenal calcium crystallization, but there are still some key issues to clarify regarding the role of THP in nephrolithiasis. By conducting a long-range follow-up of more than 250 THP-null mice and their wild-type controls, Liu et al. [58] demonstrated that renal calcification was a highly consistent phenotype of the THP-null mice. The crystals consisted primarily of CaP in the form of hydroxyapatite. They were located in the interstitial space of the renal papillae more frequently than in the tubules (particularly in older animals), and there was no accompanying inflammatory cell infiltration. The interstitial deposits of hydroxyapatite observed in THP-null mice strongly resemble the renal crystals found in human kidneys with idiopathic CaOx stones. In humans, a number of naturally occurring THP mutations are reportedly linked to autosomal dominant medullary

Protein	Role in CaOx crystallization and nephrolithiasis
Tamm-Horsfall	Inhibitor of aggregation
Osteopontin	Free OPN Inhibits crystal nucleation, growth, aggregation and attachment, immobilized OPN promotes crystal attachment
Prethrombin fragment-1	Inhibitor of growth and aggregation
Bikunin and inter-α-inhibitor	Inhibitor of nucleation, growth, aggregation and attachment
α-1-microglobulin	Inhibitor of crystallization
CD-44	Promoter of crystal attachment
Calgranulin	Inhibitor of crystal growth and aggregation
Matrix gla protein	Inhibitor of crystal deposition
Heparan sulfate	Inhibitor of crystal aggregation and attachment
Osteonectin	Calcium binding
Fibronectin	Inhibitor of crystal aggregation, attachment and endocytosis

Table 7. Crystallization-modulating macromolecules (Modified from Khan SR and Canals BK 2009 [13]).

cystic disease and familial juvenile hyperuricemic nephropathy (Uromodulin-related diseases). Mutations lead to a defective intracellular trafficking of THP, and to a reduced THP excretion and secretion. No renal stone disease has been described in patients with any of these mutations to date, however [13].

2.10. Medullary sponge kidney

Medullary nephrocalcinosis is a frequent finding in medullary sponge kidney (MSK), a renal malformation associated with renal stones, urinary acidification and concentration defects, cystic anomalies in the precalyceal ducts, a risk of urinary infections, and renal failure. In a large series of 375 patients with macroscopic nephrocalcinosis, it was found that the clinical diagnoses most frequently associated with MSK were hyperparathyroidism and dRTA [9]. The prevalence of MSK in the general population is not known because no systematic autopsy searches have been performed. In a large series of subjects undergoing iv urography for various reasons, pictures ranging from clearly evident MSK to faint radiological signs of the disease were seen in 0.5–1% of cases [59]. MSK is relatively well represented in renal stone patients, however, and has been found in up to 20% of recurrent renal calcium stone formers [60, 61].

Why this malformative condition may predispose to medullary nephrocalcinosis remains to be established. MSK is considered a rare and sporadic disorder, but a recent study showed that 50% of MSK stone formers had relatives with milder forms of MSK, suggesting that it is relatively common for MSK to be familial, and it may be inherited as an autosomal dominant trait [62]. It has also been reported that 12% of unrelated MSK patients carried in heterozygosity two very rare variants of the glial cell line-derived neurotrophic factor (GDNF) gene, and these variants were inherited and co-segregated with the MSK phenotype in some families [63].

Mezzabotta et al. [64] had the chance to conduct an *in vitro* analysis on the behavior of papillary renal cells coming from the healthy portion of a kidney resected due to renal cancer in a MSK patient with medullary nephrocalcinosis, who harbored one of these rare GDNF gene variants. They found an unexpected and previously never reported phenomenon involving the spontaneous formation of Ca_2PO_4 nodules very similar to those of calcifying vascular cells. They demonstrated that silencing the GDNF gene in a human renal cell line and cultivating the silenced cells in osteogenic conditions triggered the deposition of Ca_2PO_4. These results demonstrate the functional role of GDNF gene mutation in determining the medullary nephrocalcinosis associated with the MSK phenotype. They also provide the first experimental evidence of human renal tubular cells having a pivotal role in driving a calcification process. The role of renal cells in nephrocalcinosis is discussed in the subsequent paragraphs.

3. Proposed mechanisms of nephrocalcinosis

3.1. Tubular nephrocalcinosis

It is commonly assumed that crystals of CaOx or CaP form in the tubular fluid because of supersaturation and are presumably a renal mechanism for excreting excess waste [65–69]. In physiological conditions, this process is well controlled and lowers the risk of supersaturation [70–72]. When these control mechanisms fail, however, or changing conditions alter the solubility of the urinary calcium salts, there is a consequent crystal retention and renal calcium deposition. This may involve epithelial crystal adhesion when the crystals are smaller than the diameter of the tubular lumen or lead to crystals obstructing the tubules when crystal formation and/or aggregation becomes excessive (**Figure 5A**).

3.1.1. *Adhesion of crystals to the tubular epithelial cells: the fixed particle theory*

The first step in crystal formation is nucleation, i.e., the process by which free ions in solution become associated forming microscopic particles. Crystallization can occur in solution micro-environments, such as those potentially existing in certain parts of the nephron [73], as well as on surfaces (like those of cells), and in the extracellular matrix [74]. Nucleation is followed by an aggregation of the crystals forming in the free solution, giving rise to larger particles. Finlayson and Reid [75] postulated that crystals cannot grow large enough during the short time it takes them to transit through the tubules to be retained in the tubules because of their size ("free particle" mechanism). This led to the hypothesis that crystals can only remain in the kidney if they adhere to the tubular epithelium (the 'fixed particle' theory) [74–76]. As a general mechanism for the etiology of tubular nephrocalcinosis, it was therefore suggested that crystallization starts at particular sites on the epithelial surface, not

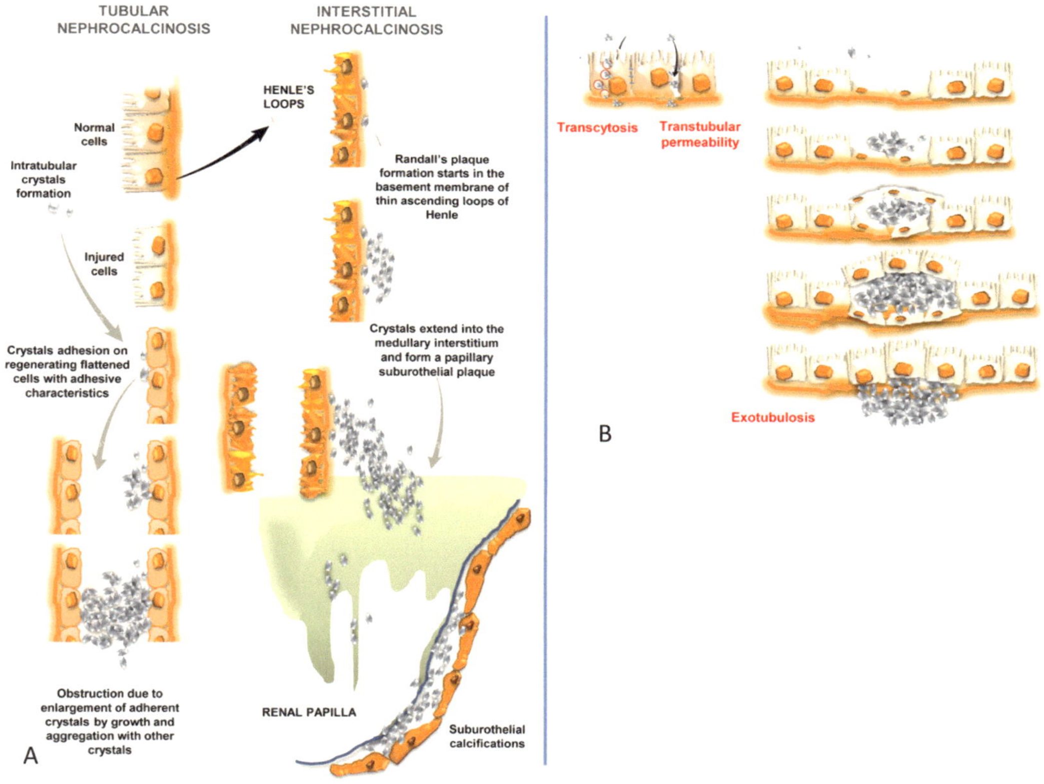

Figure 5. Proposed mechanisms of nephrocalcinosis. (A) Processes of tubular and interstitial calcium crystal deposition. (B) Possible mechanisms of interstitial crystal formation.

freely in the tubular fluid. A nascent crystal then becomes aggregated with other crystals, forming a mass large enough to occlude the nephron, leading to an obstructive tubulopathy (**Figure 5A**).

These crystals can be found in contact with the surface of injured/regenerating epithelial cells, apoptotic and/or necrotic cells, and denuded basement membranes [4, 77–84], giving the impression that the composition of the cell surface is crucial in modulating this process. In fact, it has been demonstrated on primary or immortalized tubular epithelial cells exposed to CaOx crystals that the crystal deposits preferentially adhere to injured, apoptotic, depolarized, immature, migrating, or proliferating tubular epithelial cells, rather than to fully differentiated, normal epithelia [85–88]. In this context, there is interesting evidence to suggest that proximal tubular cells bind crystals regardless of their differentiation status, whereas distal tubular cells (which are physiologically more likely to encounter crystals) only bind crystals when they are dedifferentiated [70], meaning that the distal tubular epithelium is unable to bind crystals when differentiated.

What we know about crystal adhesion in the proximal and distal tubules stems mainly from having identified the characteristics of the luminal membrane and the molecular composition of the crystal-binding epithelia, which led to the discovery of several crystal-binding molecules [4, 80, 89–93]. Importantly, these crystal-binding molecules are upregulated or redistributed to the apical membrane under certain conditions of cellular dedifferentiation, such as injury or repair, or variations in pathophysiological conditions [78, 87, 88, 94–96], which determine whether or not the crystals are retained in the kidney.

The different categories of crystal-binding molecules identified *in vitro* to date include: (i) terminal sialic acid residues [79, 97, 98]; (ii) phospholipids, i.e., phosphatidylserine [78, 84, 99, 100]; (iii) membrane-bound proteins, i.e., collagen IV [101], OPN [102–106], annexin 2 (ANX2) [107, 108] and nucleolin-related protein (NRP) [88, 93, 109]; and (iv) glycosaminoglycans, of which hyaluronan (HA) appears to be the most potent crystal-binding polysaccharide [95, 96, 110]. It has been demonstrated that other proteins, such as matrix Gla protein (MGP), are implicated in this process too [48, 111]. It is intriguing, moreover, that all known crystal-binding molecules contribute to inducing a negative cell-surface charge, a feature that has proved important in crystal adhesion to renal epithelial cells [85, 97, 112]. This would suggest that an array of aberrant phenotypes could bind crystals if there are appropriate amounts of crystals and appropriately oriented negative charges on the luminal membrane.

On the other hand, crystals and/or concomitant high concentrations of calcium, oxalate, or phosphate have been found to induce injury, proliferation, inflammatory mediator production, and oxidative stress on contact with epithelial cells *in vitro*, suggesting that epithelial dedifferentiation could be a consequence rather than a cause of crystal adhesion [113–120].

3.1.2. Is the crystal-binding cell phenotype a cause or a consequence of crystal adhesion?

Crystals do not adhere to normal epithelial cells, so it is highly unlikely that crystal adhesion might be the initial cause of cellular injury and epithelial phenotypic alterations, which are probably triggered instead by forced contact and transient interaction with normal epithelia during the passage of the crystals/oxalate. Either way, it is evident that the tubular epithelium must have a very important direct role in the initiation of intratubular nephrocalcinosis.

Some reports have suggested that the renal tubular epithelial cell injury in crystal-cell interactions occurs more easily in a setting of prior cell injury [99, 118]. The "incubation" period observed during transient toxic or mechanical crystal-cell interactions capable of affecting the tubular epithelium is consistent with the need for a shift in the epithelial phenotype prior to crystal adhesion [119–121]. This would mean that crystal adhesion is a consequence, not the initial cause of epithelial injury *in vitro*.

The nucleation of ions from the renal tubule and subsequent growth of a calcium crystal cannot usually occur and, even if it does, such processes do not proceed quickly enough to produce particles of sufficient size to be retained in the kidney, and occlude tubules simply because of their bulk [68, 76, 118, 122, 123]. The crystals are not only the outcome of the physicochemical properties and urinary concentrations of the minerals involved. They are also influenced by crystallization regulators that may promote or inhibit crystallization and by signaling pathways triggered by the crystals, thus leading to different types of renal cell injury [8, 71, 124–127]. Urine or, more properly, tubular fluid probably contains inhibitors of crystal formation that specifically prevent their nucleation, growth, or aggregation. It has been claimed that the inhibitors' role in controlling crystal formation is important in the normal defenses against the development of stones, and that abnormalities of these inhibitors may allow for stone formation and growth.

There are different types of such crystallization inhibitors in the urine, including small organic anions such as citrate, small inorganic anions such as PPis, multivalent metallic cations such as magnesium, and macromolecules such as OPN and Tamm-Horsfall protein, which can take effect on different levels during the crystal formation process (**Table 7**). Citrate lowers the saturation of CaOx by forming complexes with calcium and inhibits the aggregation of preformed crystals and the attachment of crystals to the renal epithelium [97, 128]. PPi is a substance naturally occurring in urine that has been found to inhibit the crystallization of both CaOx and CaP [129]. Magnesium has also been shown to prevent stone formation by inhibiting the growth and aggregation of crystals (and presumably interferes with their nucleation too) [130]. OPN (known to inhibit the spontaneous nucleation of crystals from solutions) was found to prevent the growth of preformed crystals in a seed growth assay [131, 132], but there is also evidence to suggest that OPN bound to the surface of cells may enhance crystal attachment [102, 103]. In addition, the inhibitory effect of OPN on CaOx aggregation *in vitro* can be switched to an aggregation promoting effect if its net negative charge is neutralized by polyarginine [133].

Tamm-Horsfall glycoprotein (THP) is the most abundant of the urinary proteins under normal circumstances [134]. THP coats CaOx crystals and prevents their adhesion to cultured epithelia, but there are few *in vivo* studies on how it would affect their aggregate, once it anchored to the epithelia [134, 135]. Another protein, called urinary prothrombin fragment 1, has been isolated from the matrix of crystals formed by adding oxalate to urine [136]. This is an effective inhibitor of CaOx crystal growth and aggregation, *in vivo* as well as *in vitro* [137].

3.2. Interstitial nephrocalcinosis

The presence of crystals in the renal interstitium is defined as interstitial nephrocalcinosis (**Figure 5A**). Although the causal role of aberrant epithelial tissue in crystal adhesion—demonstrated in renal cell lines *in vitro*, in animal models, in kidney transplant patients, and in neonates—may account for intratubular crystal formation and retention [138–140], the specific pathogenic mechanisms leading to interstitial crystal formation and deposition are still unclear [7].

Translocation of intratubular crystals and/or *de novo* interstitial calcification have been proposed as causative factors (**Figure 5B**).

3.2.1. Translocation of intratubular crystals to the interstitium

Crystal translocation can be induced by transcytosis (**Figure 5B**), a process during which small intraluminal crystals are internalized within apical vesicles (with or without the mediation of a receptor) and transferred across the cell wall to the basolateral side, where they are released into the interstitial extracellular environment [12]. Apical endocytosis of small crystals has been well described [141–144], but there is little evidence of any basolateral release of crystals into the interstitium. It has been suggested that these crystals probably disintegrate into lysosomes [142, 143, 145]. Very recently, however, Chiangjong et al. [146] demonstrated that, after exposure to CaOx crystals, renal tubular epithelial cells secrete more crystal-binding protein (enolase-1 [147]) into the basolateral compartment; the authors suggested that this protein could in turn promote CaOx crystal invasion through the renal interstitium. The translocation of crystals into the interstitium is associated with inflammation, attracting leukocytes, monocytes, and macrophages that—according to some—would then remove the crystalline material [148].

An alternative mechanism of transepithelial crystal translocation was described using the term "exotubulosis" (**Figure 5B**) in an *in vivo* study conducted by De Bruijn et al. [149, 150]. These authors demonstrated that crystals adhering to the inside wall of the tubule can be overgrown by tubular epithelial cells adjacent to the site of adhesion of the crystals. After proliferation and migration, the tubular epithelial cells cover the crystals and differentiate into a new mature epithelium, with its basement membrane on top of the crystals and its apical side directed toward the lumen, thereby restoring the epithelial integrity of the affected tubule, and translocating the crystals into the interstitium.

For a long time, translocation was the only explanation for the advent of mineral deposits in the interstitium [151, 152], but crystals can also form *de novo* in the interstitium.

3.2.2. De novo interstitial crystal formation

It has been claimed that these crystal deposits start in the interstitium around the thin limbs of the loop of Henle (below the basement membrane) and give rise to subepithelial calcifications better known as Randall's plaques [153].

Nobody knows, however, whether this *de novo* crystal formation is due merely to a chemically driven supersaturation or whether cells are involved too. For some time, the most accredited hypothesis advanced to explain the onset of interstitial nephrocalcinosis was purely physicochemical, relating to spontaneous Ca_2PO_4 crystallization in the interstitium as a result of calcium and phosphate oversaturation in this milieu. Evidence has been produced of a lower expression and defective barrier and fence functions of the tight junction in renal tubular epithelial cells exposed to CaOx crystals. This could lead to intercellular (paracellular) migration of intratubular COM crystals, and of calcium, oxalate, and phosphate ions to the interstitium to initiate tubulointerstitial injury, inflammation, and interstitial nephrocalcinosis [154–157].

Dysregulation of calcium homeostasis in the renal interstitium (and probably on a systemic level too) may have a key role in the pathogenesis of nephrocalcinosis. Bushinsky DA [154] proposed a sequence of events that could lead to an increased supersaturation and subsequent crystal formation. *"Following ingestion and absorption of dietary calcium, the renal-filtered load of calcium would increase, resulting in increased tubular calcium concentration. The medullary countercurrent mechanism would concentrate the calcium extracted from the TAL into the hypertonic papilla. The vasa recta, also with an increased calcium concentration, would fail to readily remove calcium from the interstitium. The increased serum calcium would stimulate the calcium receptor and decrease reabsorption of water in the collecting duct, further concentrating the interstitium. Vectorial proton transport into the collecting duct would alkalinize the interstitium. The pH of the vasa recta would also increase following gastric proton secretion, the so-called alkaline tide, resulting in less bicarbonate removal from the medullary interstitium. The increased pH would decrease the solubility of CaP complexes. Perhaps an extracellular matrix protein, specific to the papillary interstitium, could provide a site promoting heterogeneous nucleation, which occurs with a lower degree of supersaturation than homogeneous nucleation."*

Estimates of tubular fluid supersaturation based on data obtained in the rat suggest that CaP supersaturation often occurs in the thin limbs of the loop of Henle [158], where tubular fluid is saturated even under normal circumstances. In humans, this condition could drive the precipitation of CaP deposits at interstitial sites, in the inner medulla—known as Randall's plaques when they become extensive enough to be macroscopically visible [4, 6, 158, 159]. Randall's plaques have been proposed as a nidus for the development of the most common variety of CaOx stones [4, 160].

3.2.3. Randall's plaques

Randall demonstrated that interstitial crystals are located at, or adjacent to, the papillary tip [161]. These crystals in the papillary interstitium are composed not of CaOx (the most common solid phase found in patients with nephrolithiasis), but of CaP [162, 163], that then eroded into the urinary space, serving as a heterogeneous nucleation surface for CaOx. Randall concluded that renal stones originated as a slow deposition/crystallization of urinary salts (CaOx, CaP, uric acid) on a lesion of the renal papilla—a picture confirmed and extended in patients with idiopathic CaOx nephrolithiasis [4, 5, 164] (**Figure 6**).

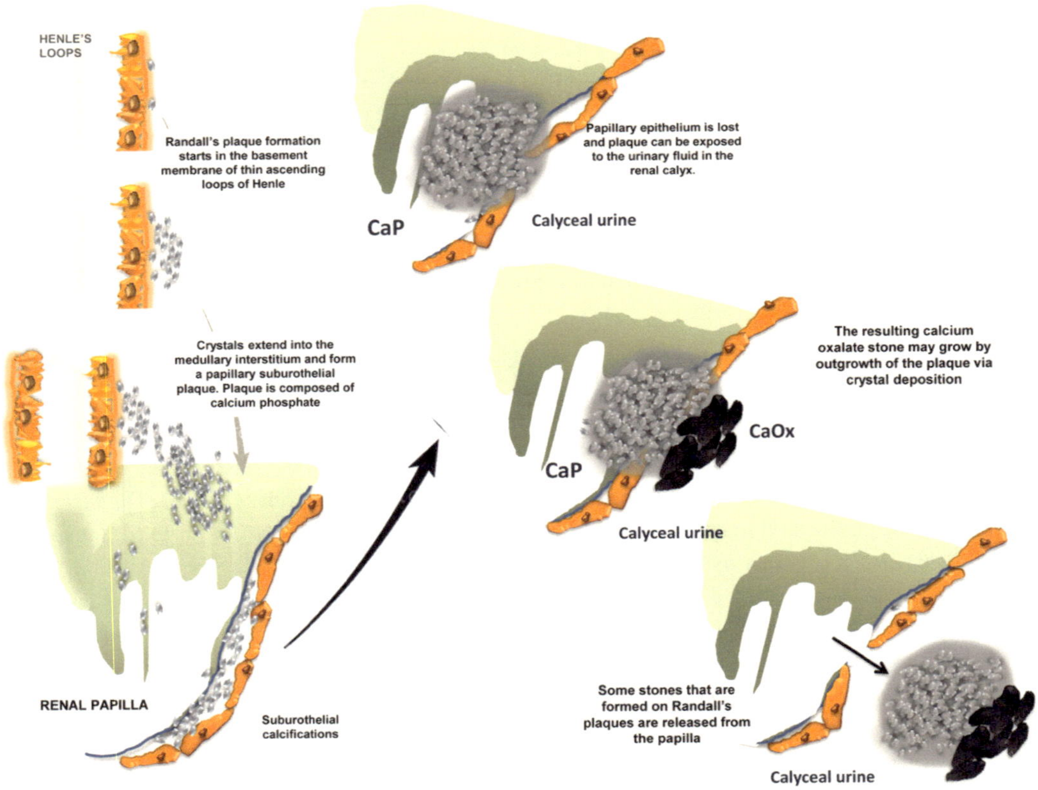

Figure 6. Mechanism of stone growing on Randall's plaque. The plaque appears in the interstitial tissue within the renal papilla, with no crystals present in any tubular lumens. The plaque is composed of calcium phosphate (CaP) in the mineral form of apatite. Papillary epithelium is lost, and the plaque can be exposed to urinary fluid in the renal calyx. The resulting calcium oxalate stone may grow and the plaque keeps the stone from flowing out with the urine, and the insolubility of the calcium oxalate makes the stone quite. Stones that are formed on Randall's plaques are released from the papilla in the renal calyx.

4. Cell-driven calcification: the example of vascular calcification

In the last decade, some researchers have attempted to clarify the effects of high oxalate and crystal concentrations on the biology of renal tubular cells because the exact role of the tubular cells in response to the influx of these potentially precipitating ions is still uncertain.

A role in the pathogenesis of Randall's plaques has also been suggested for interstitial cells capable of transdifferentiating along the bone lineage, leading to the hypothesis that nephrocalcinosis could be an osteogenic cell-driven process, similar to that of vascular calcification [64, 165–168]. Tubular epithelial cells have a well-known ability to differentiate into cells with the mesenchymal phenotype (for instance, renal interstitial myofibroblasts may originate from renal tubular cells undergoing epithelial-mesenchymal transformation) [169]. This capacity for differentiation is not exclusive to renal cells, or epithelial cells. It is shared with

Ito cells in the liver [170], and a subpopulation of smooth muscle cells (SMCs) in the intima of arteries—cell populations that are thought to be pericyte-like. Remarkably, vascular pericytes have the ability to undergo osteoblastic differentiation and mineralization [171, 172], and seem to play a crucial part in ectopic vascular calcification.

The underlying mechanisms that lead to pathological calcification are complex and thought to involve active, strictly regulated processes that are common to bone formation [54, 173, 174]. Cells that may readily undergo osteogenic-like transition include: vascular smooth muscle cells (VSMCs) [171, 175–193] in the media, myofibroblasts in the adventitia, pericytes in the microvessels [171, 172, 194], multipotent vascular mesenchymal progenitors, and valve interstitial cells [195, 196]. Vascular calcification was long thought to result from passive degeneration [197], but actually involves a complex, regulated process of biomineralization similar to osteogenesis, which mediates the deposition of bone matrix in the blood vessels [175–193].

5. Mechanisms of vascular calcification

Calcification may involve both osteogenic and chondrogenic differentiation. In humans, it is primarily osteogenic (with bone tissue formation), whereas in mice it is primarily chondrogenic (with cartilage formation). Although osteoblasts and chondroblasts are distinct cell types, they have substantial similarities in mineralization mechanisms and gene expression, leading to the formation of a complex and highly structured extracellular matrix, which can also be found in the calcified vasculature.

There is evidence to indicate that the proteins controlling bone mineralization are involved in regulating vascular calcification as well. Many key bone formation regulators and bone structural proteins, including pro-osteogenic factors like the bone morphogenetic proteins (BMP) [171–186], and inflammatory mediators such as tumor necrosis factor-α (TNF-α), are expressed in atherosclerotic plaques as well as during the osteogenic differentiation of VSMCs. These factors can induce calcification via Msx2 and Wnt signaling, which plays a crucial part in the commitment of pluripotent mesenchymal cells, activated during vascular calcification [198–202], and they have been implicated in the regulation of osteoblastic VSMC transdifferentiation [203, 204]. Wnt signaling induces an upregulated expression of the transcription factors Cfb1/Runx (core-binding factor subunit1α/runt-related transcription factor 2) and osterix [177, 178, 198–200, 205–207]. In turn, Runx2 increases the expression of the bone-related proteins osteocalcin (OCN), sclerostin, and receptor activator of nuclear factor-kappa β ligand (RANKL) [208]. Downstream from Runx2, osterix increases the expression of other bone-related proteins, including bone sialoprotein, alkaline phosphatase (ALP) [206, 209, 210], OPN [211–213], matrix γ-carboxyglutamic acid protein (MGP) [214], and osteoprotegerin (OPG) [215].

The cellular and systemic conditions that permit VSMC differentiation to osteoblast-like cells are multifactorial. At cellular level, procalcifying conditions may occur because of the factors that increase cellular stress responses. Similarly, systemic factors, such as a loss of circulating inhibitors of calcification, or changes in levels of hormonal regulators of calcium and phosphate homeostasis can also facilitate VSMC differentiation and vascular calcification.

Osteogenic differentiation of VSMCs is prevented under normal conditions by physiological inhibitors, such as MGP, OPN, and OPG [216, 217], and regulated by monocyte- and macrophage-osteoclast differentiation within the vascular wall. The growth of crystals is also hindered thermodynamically and inhibited by PPi [183, 218]. Unlike OPN, OPG, and MGP, which function in the vessel wall, fetuin A is a circulating inhibitor of calcification that has a high affinity for hydroxyapatite crystals and is thought to function by binding small CaP particles via a domain particularly rich in acidic residues, stabilizing and clearing them to phagocytes for removal [218]. *In vitro*, fetuin A inhibits the *de novo* formation of hydroxyapatite crystals, but does not affect crystals that have already formed [219]. Fetuin A also has an anti-inflammatory function, dampening the effects of CaP particles in neutrophil stimulation, and is responsible also in macrophage cytokine release and induction of apoptosis. Additionally, fetuin-A has been shown to accumulate in VSMC-derived matrix vesicles, preventing them from initiating and propagating calcification.

Given the complexity of the systems that regulate vascular calcification, it is likely that many of these factors are at work simultaneously, but in some situations the physiological balance is disrupted and vascular calcification can progress (**Figure 7**).

An alternative mechanism for vascular calcification has recently been suggested. The "circulating cell theory" [220] postulates that circulating cells coming from sources such as bone

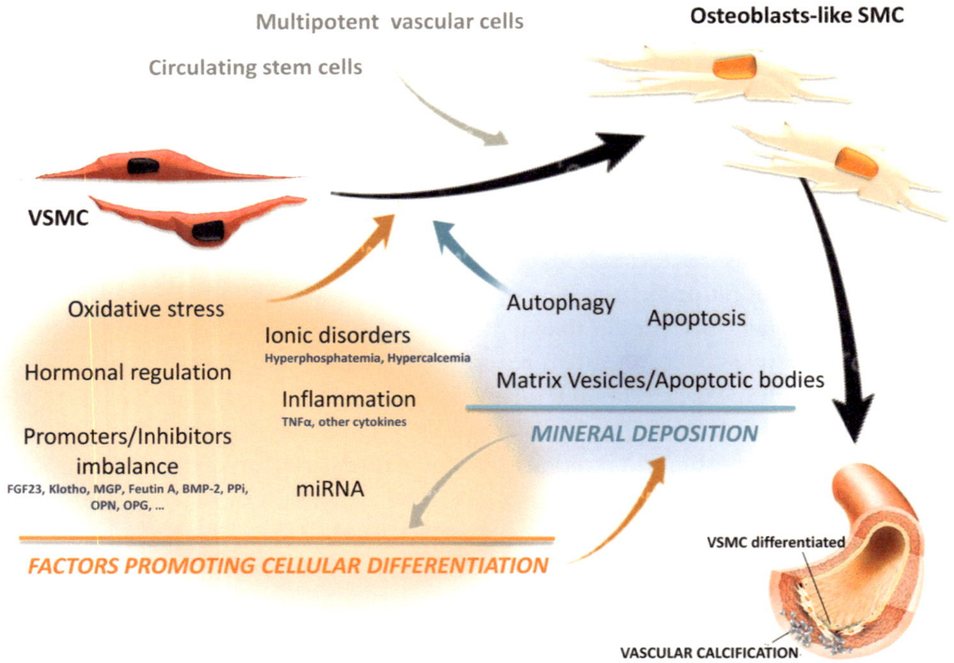

Figure 7. Physiopathological mechanisms promote cellular differentiation and mineral deposition during vascular calcification. Vascular smooth muscle cells undergo differentiation to osteoblast-like cells when exposed to different factors. These osteoblast-like cells participate in vascular calcification.

marrow may have an active role in vascular calcification. A circulating immature bone-marrow-derived cell population has been identified, and a small subset of this bone marrow population reportedly possesses bone-forming properties *in vitro*. Under the influence of chemoattractants (released by damaged endothelium, for instance), these cells may home in on diseased arteries. Under pathological conditions such as an imbalance between promoters and inhibitors of vascular calcification, this population may undergo osteogenic differentiation in the lesions, promoting vessel mineralization [220]. In another study, it has also been claimed that multipotent vascular stem cells (MVSC) in the blood vessel wall might differentiate into osteoblast-like cells [221]—though this theory remains highly controversial for the time being.

6. Factors regulating vascular calcification

6.1. Phosphate

The role of phosphate in the osteoblastic differentiation process is well established [176, 177, 181, 185, 187, 222]. *In vitro*, high extracellular phosphate concentrations induce a rise in intracellular phosphate concentrations actively mediated by three types of sodium-dependent phosphate cotransporter, of which the type III transporters Pit-1 and Pit-2 are ubiquitously expressed and predominant in humans. Only Pit-1 is required for the osteogenic differentiation of VSMCs [177, 223–225]. Increasing phosphate concentrations in the VSMCs induce their phenotypic switch to osteoblast-like cells [177, 178, 184]. In the event of renal failure, phosphate plays a key part in this mechanism [165, 168]. Vascular SMCs exposed to pro-calcifying levels of phosphate (akin to what may happen in patients with chronic kidney disease (CKD)) lose their expression of the smooth muscle contractile proteins, SM22α and SMα-actin, and express the bone markers Runx2, OPN, OCN, and ALP instead [178].

As well as phosphate, many other factors can influence the osteoblastic-like phenotype. A long-term exposure of VSMCs to a variety of chronic stresses and ionic disorders (especially hyperphosphatemia and hypercalcemia), for example, can override the action of some endogenous inhibitors, such as MGP, OPN, OPG and PPi [217], inducing differentiation [226]. Oxidative stress, inflammation, hormonal perturbations, and metabolic disorders can lead to vascular calcification too.

6.2. Oxidative stress

Oxidative stress and endoplasmic reticulum stress have both been implicated in vascular calcification and shown to promote smooth muscle cell (SMC) differentiation. In particular, oxidative stress generated in VSMCs by hyperlipidemia and oxidized lipoproteins, or a uremic milieu [227] prompts the expression of BMP2, Runx2 [228], and osterix, and governs Wnt signaling [207]. Reactive oxygen species (ROS) signaling can also induce other markers of osteoblastic differentiation. In the vascular wall, the induction of oxidative stress can recapitulate osteogenesis in the VSMC from their undifferentiated state [229]. The role of ROS formation and signaling in vascular calcification may also reveal a link between inflammation and vascular calcification, since inflammatory cytokines induce calcification via the Msx2/Wnt/β-catenin pathway [202]. It has also been found that calcium deposits colocalize with inflammatory cells both *in vitro* [230, 231] and *in vivo* [232]. Mineral crystals may therefore be pro-inflammatory per se, prompting and exacerbating the inflammation and calcification [233, 234].

6.3. Hormones

Hormones have pleiotropic effects on calcific vasculopathy. For example, the adipose-derived factor, leptin, promotes vascular cells *in vitro* [235] and *in vivo* [236], while adiponectin-deficient mice have increased levels of vascular calcification [237]. The influence of parathyroid hormone (PTH), which is involved in the bone turnover process, is also well known. PTH has a crucial role in calcium homeostasis, and so does PTH-related peptide (PTHrP), and the two may function as pathological calcification mediators. Both PTH and PTHrP prevent VSMC calcification in a dose-dependent manner by inhibiting ALP activity [238]. In addition, PTHrP is secreted from VSMCs, an action that is impaired by calcitriol (1,25-dihydroxyvitamin D, the active form of vitamin D) [239]. PTH not only promotes the release of calcium from bone but also mobilizes salts, including bicarbonate and phosphate and impairs renal phosphate excretion, leading, for example, to advanced nephron loss in CKD patients, and thus resulting in severe hyperphosphatemia [240]. Accrued high levels of serum phosphate then further stimulate the secretion of PTH, forming a vicious cycle [241]. Hyperphosphatemia increases FGF23 (a protein released by bone), which—together with its co-receptor Klotho (a transmembrane protein expressed by the kidney and blood vessels)—may also be a pathogenic factor in vascular calcification [242, 243]. Klotho maintains the balance of circulating calcium and phosphate [244]. Activation of the vitamin D receptor increases the expression of Klotho and FGF23 to promote renal phosphate excretion by downregulating the sodium phosphate transporters Slc34A1/NaPi-2a and Slc34A3/NaPi-2c. Intriguingly, Klotho inhibits vascular calcification by preventing VSMC differentiation while disrupting Klotho-FGF23 signaling results in hyperphosphatemia with ectopic calcification [244, 245].

Calcitriol may also exacerbate dystrophic calcification. Vitamin D toxicity is a common animal model used to study vascular calcification [246]. Calcitriol dose-dependently increases both calcification and ALP activity in VSMCs [239]. In response to interferon-γ, macrophages express 25-hydroxyvitamin D 1α-hydroxylase, the enzyme needed to convert 25-hydroxyvitamin D into calcitriol [239]. Once calcitriol binds to its receptor, signaling through this pathway has pleiotropic effects. The vitamin D receptor influences many genes in the vessel wall, including vascular endothelial growth factor (VEGF), matrix metalloproteinase 9, myosin, and structural proteins (including elastin and type I collagen [247–250], and this explains some of the effects of calcitriol on vascular calcification.

Glucocorticoids, a class of steroid hormones with anti-inflammatory properties, have also been shown to mediate osteoblastic differentiation and thereby promote ectopic calcification. Long-term glucocorticoid use has been associated with osteoporosis, however, and these compounds have been shown to initiate differentiation to an osteochondrogenic phenotype in vascular cells [251, 252]. Similarly, pericytes exposed to dexamethasone exhibit a weaker expression of MGP and OPN, and an increased ALP activity and calcium deposition.

6.4. Matrix vesicles

Bone formation involves hydroxyapatite [$Ca_{10}(PO_4)_6(OH)_2$] crystals, which begin to develop matrix vesicles that grow out of osteoblasts. VSMC that have undergone osteoblastic differentiation are able to release similar mineralization-competent matrix vesicle-like structures in the extracellular matrix too [176, 180, 215, 226, 253–256]. These matrix vesicles serve as mineral nucleation sites and are responsible for the initial deposition of calcium and phosphate in blood vessels (**Figure 7**). Matrix vesicles contain proteins related to calcification, extracellular matrix and extracellular matrix-modifying enzymes, calcium channels, trafficking and cytoskeletal proteins, oxidant and endoplasmic stress-related proteins, and other serum proteins [226]. All these proteins are involved in the disruption of the normal vessel architecture and thus serve as the nidus for calcification. Matrix vesicles also have an increased expression and activity of transglutaminase 2, a calcium-dependent enzyme that promotes extracellular matrix crosslinking, and matrix metalloproteinase-2 [226, 257]. Matrix vesicles are secreted from multivesicular bodies and are enriched with exosomes found to contain amorphous calcium-phosphate crystals under calcifying conditions, and detected at the site of calcification [258].

Prolonged cellular stress may activate homeostatic repair processes, or cells may undergo apoptosis when overwhelmed by the stress. Apoptosis regulates VSMC calcification *in vitro* and inhibiting apoptosis reduces VSMC calcification [171, 176, 259–261]. In advanced carotid atherosclerotic plaques, the matrix vesicles contain high levels of BAX (a pro-apoptotic member of the BCL2 family), indicating that they may be remnants of apoptotic cells [171, 176, 260]. Apoptotic VSMC-derived matrix vesicle-like structures are also able to concentrate and crystallize calcium, triggering calcification [176, 183, 189, 193, 222]. It has likewise been reported that chondrocyte-derived apoptotic bodies might contribute to the calcification of articular cartilage [262]. All these data support the idea that the formation of apoptotic bodies may be another factor initiating ectopic calcification in cells under certain conditions.

Autophagy—a catabolic process that may be an adaptive response to cell stress—has been found to limit SMC calcification by inhibiting matrix vesicle release. When phosphate levels are high, inhibiting autophagy resulted in an increased VSMC calcium deposition. Downregulating autophagy was also associated with a loss of VSMC contractile proteins, but not with any VSMC differentiation to an osteogenic phenotype. On the other hand, inhibiting autophagy did increase the release of procalcific matrix vesicles with high levels of ALP activity [263]. In short, factors that interfere with autophagy are likely to increase VSMC and vascular calcification.

6.5. MicroRNAs

MicroRNAs (miRs) have emerged as key regulators of cell differentiation to osteoblast-like cells, regulating gene expression under pro-calcifying conditions. Some studies have described a stronger expression of miRs targeting smooth muscle contractile proteins and a weaker expression of miRs targeting osteoblast differentiation markers under these conditions [264]. For example, the miR-143/145 complex, which regulates the expression of VSMC differentiation markers and Kruppel-like factor4 (KLF4), is downregulated; and KLF4 is known to control bone homeostasis by negatively regulating both osteoclast and osteoblast differentiation [265]. Other studies showed that downregulation of miR-204, miR-205, miR-133a, or miR-30b/c in VSMCs occurs prior to calcification and upregulates Runx2 expression [266, 267]. Micro-RNA-125b, which targets Ets1 and osterix, was found downregulated 21 days after exposing VSMCs to osteogenic medium [268]. Another set of miRs, miR-135a(*n*), miR-762, miR-714, miR-712(*n*), that target the calcium flux proteins NCX1, PMCA1, and NCKX4, have also been implicated in VSMC calcification [266]. It is still not clear, however, whether these miRs are really important in VSMC differentiation to an osteoblast-like phenotype, or whether this process is associated with changes in the expression of a panel of miRs targeting several proteins important for calcification.

7. Evidence of cell-driven renal calcification

It is worth considering the possibility of ectopic renal calcification being an osteogenic-like process. Evidence to support the notion that resident renal cells could be prompted to transdifferentiate, or differentiate along an osteogenic lineage, comes from the following observations. Madin-Darby canine kidney (MDCK) cells grown in monolayers directly on a plastic dish, or a dish coated with collagen gel, developed small blisters/domes/nodules after 21 days that became more prominent after 30 days [269, 270]. Microscopic examination showed that the nodules were CaP crystals. MDCK cells grown in agar produced spherical colonies in which layers of epithelial cells, with their apical surface on the outside, enclosed CaP crystal deposits on the basal side of the epithelium [90, 93, 270–272].

Kumar et al. [71] found that rat inner medullary collecting duct cells grown in a calcifying medium formed calcifying nodules that were positive for typical bone proteins. Miyazawa et al. [273, 274] reported finding that CaOx crystals upregulated vimentin (VIM) in normal rat kidney proximal cells and that other genes, such as OPN, fibronectin (FN), cathepsins B and L, and mitogen-activated protein kinase, related to the pathogenesis of stone formation. Using MDCK cells grown for 28 days in the presence of 10 mM β-glycerophosphate, Azari et al. identified a mineralization process with an increased ALP activity and the presence of small aggregates of hydroxyapatite crystals within membrane-bounded vesicles [275]. Other related osteogenic genes (RUNX1 and 2, osterix, BMP2 and 7, bone morphogenetic protein receptor 2, collagen, OCN, osteonectin (ON), OPN, MGP, OPG, cadherins, FN, and VIM) were found upregulated in the kidney of hyperoxaluric rats [276, 277]. Khan et al., again, showed a pronounced expression of MGP, together with that of collagen, OPN and FN, in renal medullary peritubular vessels of hyperoxaluric rats [111], confirming that the tubular epithelial cells of hyperoxaluric kidneys acquired a number of osteoblastic features, and suggesting a dedifferentiation of epithelial cells to the osteogenic phenotype [278].

Mezzabotta et al. were the first to provide evidence of human renal cells transdifferentiating into an osteogenic-like phenotype, producing CaP deposits [64]. They found spontaneous instances of calcification phenomena in primary papillary renal cells derived from a patient with medullary sponge kidney (MSK) and medullary nephrocalcinosis, who carried a mutation in the GDNF gene. To investigate whether this spontaneous mineralization was merely a physicochemical phenomenon or a well-organized biomineralization process, they searched for any sign of the bone mineralization machinery being expressed in the cells. They found the cells positive for osteogenic markers such as ON, ALP, collagen I, laminin and Runx2, and weakly positive for OCN, but negative for OPN (a known inhibitor of crystal formation). The upregulation of ON and downregulation of OPN were also demonstrated at mRNA level. Investigating which cells were the main actors behind the phenomenon observed, the authors found that the cells were mesenchymal stroma cells (MSCs), which are very similar to pericytes. The microvasculature of the renal papilla is particularly rich in pericytes, which regulate microvascular integrity in the peritubular capillary network and give the descending vasa recta its contractile function [279]. Thus, like VSMCs, papillary MSCs associated with the perivascular niche may be capable of driving an osteogenic process under certain conditions.

In the same paper, the Authors demonstrated that human renal tubular HK-2 cells exposed to an osteogenic medium displayed the ability to produce Ca_2PO_4 by regulating the ON/OPN ratio in favor of ON.

Overall, all these very interesting data underscore that renal cells may acquire an osteoblast-like phenotype, and that a process very similar to vascular calcification may have a role in the development of human nephrocalcinosis.

Author details

Giovanna Priante, Monica Ceol, Liliana Terrin, Lisa Gianesello, Federica Quaggio, Dorella Del Prete and Franca Anglani*

*Address all correspondence to: franca.anglani@unipd.it

Laboratory of Histomorphology and Molecular Biology of the Kidney, Nephrology Unit, Department of Medicine DIMED, University of Padua, Padua, Italy

References

[1] Saigal CS, Joyce G, Timilsina AR. Urologic Diseases in America project. Direct and indirect costs of nephrolithiasis in an employed population: Opportunity for disease management. Kidney International. 2005;**68**:1808-1814

[2] Gambaro G, Vezzoli G, Casari G Rampoldi L, D'Angelo A, Borghi L. Genetics of hypercalciuria and calcium nephrolithiasis: From the rare monogenic to the common polygenic forms. American Journal of Kidney Diseases. 2004;**44**:963-986

[3] Worcester EM, Coe FL. Nephrolithiasis. Primary Care. 2008;**35**:369-391

[4] Evan AP, Lingeman JE, Coe FL Parks JH, Bledsoe SB, Shao Y, Sommer AJ, Paterson RF, Kuo RL, Grynpas M. Randall's plaque of patients with nephrolithiasis begins in basement membranes of thin loops of Henle. Journal of Clinical Investigation. 2003;**111**:607-616

[5] Evan AP, Coe FL, Lingeman JE, Shao Y, Sommer AJ, Bledsoe SB, Anderson JC, Worcester EM. Mechanisms of formation of human calcium oxalate renal stones on Randall's plaque. The Anatomical Record (Hoboken.). 2007;**290**:1315-1323

[6] Sayer JA, Carr G, Simmons NL. Nephrocalcinosis: Molecular insights into calcium precipitation within the kidney. Clinical Science (London). 2004;**106**:549-561

[7] Shavit L, Jaeger P, Unwin RJ. What is nephrocalcinosis? Kidney International. 2015;**88**:35-43

[8] Oliveira B, Kleta R, Bockenhauer D, Walsh SB. Genetic, pathophysiological, and clinical aspects of nephrocalcinosis. American Journal of Physiology Renal Physiology. 2016;**311**:F1243-F1252

[9] Wrong O. Nephrocalcinosis. In: Davison AM, Camerun JS, Grunfeld JP, Ponticelli C, Van Ypersele C, Ritz E, Winearls C, editors. Oxford Textbook of Clinical Nephrology. Oxford: Oxford University Press; 2005. p. 1375

[10] Schepens D, Verswijvel G, Kuypers D, Vanrenterghem Y. Images in nephrology. Renal cortical nephrocalcinosis. Nephrology Dialysis Transplantation. 2000;**15**:1080-1082

[11] Lloyd Thomas HG, Balme RH, Key JJ. Tram line calcification in RCN. British Medical Journal. 1962;**1**:909-911

[12] Kumar V, Farell G, Yu S, Harrington S, Fitzpatrick L, Rzewuska E, Miller VM, Lieske JC. Cell biology of pathologic renal calcification: Contribution of crystal transcytosis, cell-mediated calcification, and nanoparticles. Journal of Investigative Medicine. 2006;**54**:412-424

[13] Khan SR, Canales BK. Genetic basis of renal cellular dysfunction and the formation of kidney stones. Urological Research. 2009;**37**:169-180

[14] Dimke H, Hoenderop JG, Bindels RJ. Hereditary tubular transport disorders: Implications for renal handling of Ca2+ and Mg2+. Clinical Science (London). 2009;**118**:1-18

[15] Friedman PA, Gesek FA. Cellular calcium transport in renal epithelia: Measurement, mechanisms, and regulation. Physiological Reviews. 1995;**75**:429-471

[16] Coe FL, Worcester EM, Evan AP. Idiopathic hypercalciuria and formation of calcium renal stones. Nature Reviews Nephrology. 2016;**12**:519-533

[17] Moe OW, Bonny O. Genetic hypercalciuria. Journal of the American Society of Nephrology. 2005;**16**:729-745

[18] Wagner CA, Rubio-Aliaga I, Biber J, Hernando N. Genetic diseases of renal phosphate handling. Nephrology Dialysis Transplantation. 2014;**29**(Suppl 4):iv45-iv54

[19] Soleimani M. SLC26 Cl-/HCO3- exchangers in the kidney: Roles in health and disease. Kidney International. 2013;**84**:657-666

[20] Hoppe B. An update on primary hyperoxaluria. Nature Reviews Nephrology. 2012;**8**: 467-475

[21] Gee HY, Jun I, Braun DA, Lawson JA, Halbritter J, Shril S, Nelson CP, Tan W, Stein D, Wassner AJ, Ferguson MA, Gucev Z, Sayer JA, Milosevic D, Baum M, Tasic V, Lee MG, Hildebrandt F. Mutations in SLC26A1 cause nephrolithiasis. American Journal of Human Genetics. 2016;**98**:1228-1234

[22] Lu X, Sun D, Xu B, Pan J, Wei Y, Mao X, Yu D, Liu H, Gao B. In silico screening and molecular dynamic study of non synonymous single nucleotide polymorphisms associated with kidney stones in the SLC26A6 gene. Journal of Urology. 2016;**196**:118-123

[23] Hamm LL. Renal handling of citrate. Kidney International. 1990;**38**:728-735

[24] Zuckerman JM, Assimos DG. Hypocitraturia: Pathophysiology and medical management. Reviews in Urology. 2009;**11**:134-144

[25] Ohana E, Shcheynikov N, Moe OW, Muallem S. SLC26A6 and NaDC-1 transporters interact to regulate oxalate and citrate homeostasis. Journal of the American Society of Nephrology. 2013;**24**:1617-1626

[26] Mossetti G, Vuotto P, Rendina D, Numis FG, Viceconti R, Giordano F, Cioffi M, Scopacasa F, Nunziata V. Association between vitamin D receptor gene polymorphisms and tubular citrate handling in calcium nephrolithiasis. Journal of Internal Medicine. 2003;**253**:194-200

[27] Okamoto N, Aruga S, Matsuzaki S, Takahashi S, Matsushita K, Kitamura T. Associations between renal sodium-citrate cotransporter (hNaDC-1) gene polymorphism and urinary citrate excretion in recurrent renal calcium stone formers and normal controls. International Journal of Urology. 2007;**14**:344-349

[28] Rendina D, De Filippo G, Gianfrancesco F, Muscariello R, Schiano di Cola M, Strazzullo P, Esposito T. Evidence for epistatic interaction between VDR and SLC13A2 genes in the pathogenesis of hypocitraturia in recurrent calcium oxalate stone formers. Journal of Nephrology. 2017;**30**:411-418

[29] Shah O, Assimos DG, Holmes RP. Genetic and dietary factors in urinary citrate excretion. Journal of Endourology. 2005;**19**:177-182

[30] Hess B, Hasler-Strub U, Ackermann D, Jaeger P. Metabolic evaluation of patients with recurrent idiopathic calcium nephrolithiasis. Nephrology Dialysis Transplantation. 1997;**12**:1362-1368

[31] Konrad M, Schlingmann KP. Inherited disorders of renal hypomagnesaemia. Nephrology Dialysis Transplantation. 2014;**29**(Suppl 4):iv63-iv71

[32] Naderi AS, Reilly Jr RF. Hereditary etiologies of hypomagnesemia. Nature Clinical Practice Nephrology. 2008;**4**:80-89

[33] Sidhu H, Gupta R, Thind SK, Nath R. Inhibition of calcium oxalate monohydrate (COM) crystal growth by pyrophosphate, citrate and rat urine. Urological Research. 1986;**14**:299-303

[34] Grases F, Ramis M, Costa-Bauzá A. Effects of phytate and pyrophosphate on brushite and hydroxyapatite crystallization. Comparison with the action of other polyphosphates. Urological Research. 2000;**28**:136-140

[35] Laminski NA, Meyers AM, Sonnekus MI, Smyth AE. Prevalence of hypocitraturia and hypopyrophosphaturia in recurrent calcium stone formers: As isolated defects or associated with other metabolic abnormalities. Nephron. 1990;**56**:379-386

[36] Moochhala SH. Extracellular pyrophosphate in the kidney: How does it get there and what does it do? Nephron Physiology. 2012;**120**:33-38

[37] Carr G, Sayer JA, Simmons NL. Expression and localization of the pyrophosphate transporter, ANK, in murine kidney cells. Cellular Physiology and Biochemistry. 2007;**20**: 507-516

[38] Ho AM, Johnson MD, Kingsley DM. Role of the mouse ank gene in control of tissue calcification and arthritis. Science. 2000;**289**:265-270

[39] Mitton-Fitzgerald E, Gohr CM, Bettendorf B, Rosenthal AK. The role of ANK in calcium pyrophosphate deposition disease. Current Rheumatology Reports. 2016;**18**:25

[40] Kurtz I. Molecular mechanisms and regulation of urinary acidification. Comprehensive Physiology. 2014;**4**:1737-1774

[41] Roy A, Al-bataineh MM, Pastor-Soler NM. Collecting duct intercalated cell function and regulation. Clinical Journal of the American Society of Nephrology. 2015;**10**:305-324

[42] Batlle D, Haque SK. Genetic causes and mechanisms of distal renal tubular acidosis. Nephrology Dialysis Transplantation. 2012;**27**:3691-3704

[43] Haque SK, Ariceta G, Batlle D. Proximal renal tubular acidosis: A not so rare disorder of multiple etiologies. Nephrology Dialysis Transplantation. 2012;**27**:4273-4287

[44] Santos F, Gil-Peña H, Alvarez-Alvarez S. Renal tubular acidosis. Current Opinion in Pediatrics. 2017;**29**:206-210

[45] Kurtz I, Zhu Q. Structure, function, and regulation of the SLC4 NBCe1 transporter and its role in causing proximal renal tubular acidosis. Current Opinion in Nephrology and Hypertension. 2013;**22**:572-583

[46] Fry AC, Karet FE. Inherited renal acidoses. Physiology (Bethesda). 2007;**22**:202-211

[47] Mohebbi N, Ferraro PM, Gambaro G, Unwin R. Tubular and genetic disorders associated with kidney stones. Urolithiasis. 2017;**45**:127-137

[48] Khan SR, Kok DJ. Modulators of urinary stone formation. Frontiers in Bioscience. 2004;**9**: 1450-1482

[49] Rimer JD, Kolbach-Mandel AM, Ward MD, Wesson JA. The role of macromolecules in the formation of kidney stones. Urolithiasis. 2017;**45**:57-74

[50] 93. Korkmaz C, Ozcan A, Akcar N. Increased frequency of ultrasonographic findings suggestive of renal stone patients with ankolysing spondylitis. Clinical and Experimental Rheumatology. 2005;**23**:389-392

[51] Min W, Sgiraga H, Chalko C, Goldfarb S, Krishna GG, Hoyer JR. Quantitative studies of human urinary excretion of uropontin. Kidney International. 1998;**53**:189-193

[52] Fisher LW, Hawkins GR, Tuross N, Termine JD. Purification and partial characterization of small proteoglycans I and II, bone sialoproteins I and II, and osteonectin from the mineral compartment of developing human bone. The Journal of Biological Chemistry. 1987;**262**:9702-9708

[53] Singh K, DeVouge MW, Mukherjee BB. Physiological properties and differential glycosylation of phosphorylated and non phosphorylated forms of osteopontin secreted by normal rat kidney cells. The Journal of Biological Chemistry. 1990;**265**:18696-18701

[54] Paloian NJ, Leaf EM, Giachelli CM. Osteopontin protects against high phosphate-induced nephrocalcinosis and vascular calcification. Kidney International. 2016;**89**:1027-1036

[55] Safarinejad MR, Shafiei N, Safarinejad S. Association between polymorphisms in osteopontin gene (SPP1) and first episode calcium oxalate urolithiasis. Urolithiasis. 2013;**41**:303-313

[56] Arcidiacono T, Mingione A, Macrina L, Pivari F, Soldati L, Vezzoli G. Idiopathic calcium nephrolithiasis: A review of pathogenic mechanisms in the light of genetic studies. American Journal of Nephrology. 2014;**40**:499-506

[57] Gao B, Yasui T, Itoh Y, Li Z, Okada A, Tozawa K, Hayashi Y, Kohri K. Association of osteopontin gene haplotypes with nephrolithiasis. Kidney International. 2007;**72**:592-598

[58] Liu Y, Mo L, Goldfarb DS, Evan AP, Liang F, Khan SR, Lieske JC, Wu XR. Progressive renal papillary calcification and ureteral stone formation in mice deficient for Tamm-Horsfall protein. American Journal of Physiology Renal Physiology. 2010;**299**:F469-F478

[59] Palubinskas AJ. Renal pyramidal structure opacification in excretory urography and its relation to Medullary Sponge Kidney. Radiology. 1963;**81**:963-970

[60] Thomas E, Witte Y, Thomas J, Arvis G. Cacchi and Ricci's disease. Radiology, epidemiology and biology. Progres en Urologie. 2000;**10**:29-35

[61] Gambaro G, Feltrin GP, Lupo A, Bonfante L, D'Angelo A, Antonello A. Medullary sponge kidney (Lenarduzzi-Cacchi-Ricci disease): A Padua Medical School discovery in the 1930s. Kidney International. 2006;**69**:663-670

[62] Fabris A, Lupo A, Ferraro PM, Anglani F, Pei Y, Danza FM, Gambaro G. Familial clustering of medullary sponge kidney is autosomal dominant with reduced penetrance and variable expressivity. Kidney International. 2013;**83**:272-277

[63] Torregrossa R, Anglani F, Fabris A, Gozzini A, Tanini A, Del Prete D, Cristofaro R, Artifoni L, Abaterusso C, Marchionna N, Lupo A, D'Angelo A, Gambaro G. Identification of GDNF gene sequence variations in patients with medullary sponge kidney disease. Clinical Journal of the American Society of Nephrology. 2010;**5**:1205-1210

[64] Mezzabotta F, Cristofaro R, Ceol M, Del Prete D, Priante G, Familiari A, Fabris A, D'Angelo A, Gambaro G, Anglani F. Spontaneous calcification process in primary renal cells from a medullary sponge kidney patient harbouring a GDNF mutation. Journal of Cellular and Molecular Medicine. 2015;**19**:889-902

[65] Kok DJ. Crystallization and stone formation inside the nephron. Scanning Microscopy. 1996;**10**:471-484

[66] Asplin JR, Parks JH,Coe FL. Dependence of upper limit of metastability on supersaturation in nephrolithiasis. Kidney International. 1997;**52**:1602-1608

[67] Ryall RL, Fleming DE, Grover PK, Chauvet M, Dean CJ, Marshall VR. The hole truth: Intracrystalline proteins and calcium oxalate kidney stones. Molecular Urology. 2000;**4**: 391-402

[68] Ryall RL. Macromolecules and urolithiasis: Parallels and paradoxes. Nephron Physiology. 2004;**98**:37-42

[69] Verkoelen CF, Verhulst A. Proposed mechanisms in renal tubular crystal retention. Kidney International. 2007;**72**:13-18

[70] Verkoelen CF, Van Der Boom BG, Kok DJ Houtsmuller AB, Visser P, Schröder FH, Romijn JC. Cell type-specific acquired protection from crystal adherence by renal tubule cells in culture. Kidney International. 1999;**55**:1426-1433

[71] Kumar V, Peña de la Vega L, Farell G, Lieske JC. Urinary macromolecular inhibition of crystal adhesion to renal epithelial cells is impaired in male stone formers. Kidney International. 2005;**68**:1784-1792

[72] Hebert SC. Extracellular calcium-sensing receptor: Implications for calcium and magnesium handling in the kidney. Kidney International. 1996;**50**:2129-2139

[73] Olszta MJ, Odom DJ, Douglas EP, Gower LB. A new paradigm for biomineral formation: Mineralization via an amorphous liquid-phase precursor. Connective Tissue Research. 2003;**44**(Suppl 1):326-333

[74] Lieske JC, Hammes MS, Toback FG. Role of calcium oxalate monohydrate crystal interactions with renal epithelial cells in the pathogenesis of nephrolithiasis: A review. Scanning Microscopy. 1998;**10**:519-534

[75] Finlayson B, Reid F. The expectation of free and fixed particles in urinary stone disease. Investigative Urology. 1978;**15**:442-448

[76] Kok DJ, Khan SR. Calcium oxalate nephrolithiasis, a free or fixed particle disease. Kidney International. 1994;**46**:847-854

[77] Khan SR. Calcium oxalate crystal interaction with renal tubular epithelium, mechanism of crystal adhesion and its impact on stone development. Urological Research. 1995;**23**:71-79

[78] Bigelow MW, Wiessner JH, Kleinman JG, Mandel NS. Surface exposure of phosphatidylserine increases calcium oxalate crystal attachment to IMCD cells. American Journal of Physiology. 1997;**272**:F55-F62

[79] Verkoelen CF, Van Der Boom BG, Kok DJ Romijn JC. Sialic acid and crystal binding. Kidney International. 2000;**57**:1072-1082

[80] Lieske JC, Toback FG, Deganello S. Sialic acid-containing glycoproteins on renal cells determine nucleation of calcium oxalate dehydrate crystals. Kidney International. 2001;**60**:1784-1791

[81] Asselman M, Verhulst A, De Broe ME Verkoelen CF. Calcium oxalate crystal adherence to hyaluronan-, osteopontin-, and CD44-expressing injured/regenerating tubular epithelial cells in rat kidneys. Journal of the American Society of Nephrology. 2003;**14**:3155-3166

[82] Khan SR, Finlayson B, Hackett RL. Histologic study of the early events in oxalate induced intranephronic calculosis. Investigative Urology. 1979;**3**:199-202

[83] Dykstra MJ, Hackett RL. Ultrastructural events in early calcium oxalate crystal formation in rats. Kidney International. 1979;**6**:640-650

[84] Sarica K, Erbagci A, Yagci F Bakir K, Erturhan S, Uçak R. Limitation of apoptotic changes in renal tubular cell injury induced by hyperoxaluria. Urological Research. 2004;**32**:271-277

[85] Riese RJ, Mandel NS, Wiessner JH, Mandel GS, Becker CG, Kleinman JG. Cell polarity and calcium oxalate crystal adherence to cultured collecting duct cells. American Journal of Physiology. 1992;262(**2 Pt 2**):F177-F184

[86] Bigelow MW, Wiessner JH, Kleinman JG, Mandel NS. Calcium oxalate crystal attachment to cultured kidney epithelial cell lines. Journal of Urology. 1998;**4**:1528-1532

[87] Verhulst A, Asselman M, Persy VP, Schepers MS, Helbert MF, Verkoelen CF, De Broe ME. Crystal retention capacity of cells in the human nephron: Involvement of CD44 and its ligands hyaluronic acid and osteopontin in the transition of a crystal binding-into a nonadherent epithelium. Journal of the American Society of Nephrology. 2003;**1**:107-115

[88] Kleinman JG, Sorokina EA, Wesson JA (2010) Induction of apoptosis with cisplatin enhances calcium oxalate crystal adherence to inner medullary collecting duct cells. Urological Research. 2010;**38**:97-104

[89] Vervaet BA, D'Haese PC, De Broe ME, Verhulst A. Crystalluric and tubular epithelial parameters during the onset of intratubular nephrocalcinosis: Illustration of the 'fixed particle' theory in vivo. Nephrology Dialysis Transplantation. 2009;**24**:3659-3668

[90] Lieske JC, Toback FG, Deganello S. Direct nucleation of calcium oxalate dihydrate crystals onto the surface of living renal epithelial cells in culture. Kidney International. 1998;**54**:796-803

[91] Ratkalkar VN, Kleinman JG. Mechanisms of stone formation. Clinical Reviews in Bone and Mineral Metabolism. 2011;**9**:187-197

[92] Geiger B, Volk T, Volberg T, Bendori R. Molecular interactions in adherans-type contacts. Journal of Cell Science. 1987;**8**(Suppl):251-272

[93] Lieske JC, Toback FG. Renal cell-urinary crystal interactions. Current Opinion in Nephrology and Hypertension. 2000;**9**:349-355

[94] Sorokina EA, Wesson JA, Kleinman JG. An acidic peptide sequence of nucleolin-related protein can mediate the attachment of calcium oxalate to renal tubule cells. Journal of the American Society of Nephrology. 2004;**8**:2057-2065

[95] Verkoelen CF, van der Boom BG, Romijn JC. Identification of hyaluronan as a crystal-binding molecule at the surface of migrating and proliferating MDCK cells. Kidney International. 2000;**3**:1045-1054

[96] Asselman M, Verhulst A, Van Ballegooijen ES, Bangma CH, Verkoelen CF, De Broe ME. Hyaluronan is apically secreted and expressed by proliferating or regenerating renal tubular cells. Kidney International. 2005;**1**:71-83

[97] Lieske JC, Leonard R, Swift H, Toback FG. Adhesion of calcium oxalate monohydrate crystals to anionic sites on the surface of renal epithelial cells. American Journal of Physiology. 1996;**270**:F192-F199

[98] Lieske JC, Norris R, Toback FG. Adhesion of hydroxyapatite crystals to anionic sites on the surface of renal epithelial cells. American Journal of Physiology. 1997;**273**:F224-F233

[99] Wiessner JH, Hasegawa AT, Hung LY, Mandel GS, Mandel NS. Mechanisms of calcium oxalate crystal attachment to injured renal collecting duct cells. Kidney International. 2001;**2**:637-644

[100] Cao LC, Jonassen J, Honeyman TW Scheid C. Oxalate-induced redistribution of phosphatidylserine in renal epithelial cells: Implications for kidney stone disease. American Journal of Physiology. 2001;**21**:69-77

[101] Kohri K, Kodama M, Ishikawa Y, Katayama Y, Matsuda H, Imanishi M, Takada M, Katoh Y, Kataoka K, Akiyama T. Immunofluorescent study on the interaction between collagen and calcium oxalate crystals in the renal tubules. European Urology. 1991;**3**:249-252

[102] Yamate T, Kohri K, Umekawa T, Amasaki N, Amasaki N, Isikawa Y, Iguchi M, Kurita T. The effect of osteopontin on the adhesion of calcium oxalate crystals to Madin-Darby canine kidney cells. European Urology. 1996;**3**:388-393

[103] Yamate T, Kohri K, Umekawa T, Iguchi M, Kurita T. Osteopontin antisense oligonucleotide inhibits adhesion of calcium oxalate crystals in Madin-Darby canine kidney cell. Journal of Urology. 1998;**4**:1506-1512

[104] Yamate T, Kohri K, Umekawa T, Konya E, Ishikawa Y, Iguchi M, Kurita T. Interaction between osteopontin on Madin-Darby canine kidney cell membrane and calcium oxalate crystal. Urologia Internationalis. 1999;**2**:81-86

[105] Wesson JA, Johnson RJ, Mazzali M, Beshensky AM, Stietz S, Giachelli C, Liaw L, Alpers CE, Couser WG, Kleinman JG, Hughes J. Osteopontin is a critical inhibitor of calcium oxalate crystal formation and retention in renal tubules. Journal of the American Society of Nephrology. 2003;**14**:139-147

[106] Mo L, Liaw L, Evan AP, Sommer AJ, Lieske JC, Wu XR. Renal calcinosis and stone formation in mice lacking osteopontin, Tamm-Horsfall protein, or both. American Journal of Physiology Renal Physiology. 2007;**293**:F1935-F1943

[107] Kumar V, Farell G, Deganello S, Lieske JC. Annexin II is present on renal epithelial cells and binds calcium oxalate monohydrate crystals. Journal of the American Society of Nephrology. 2003;**2**:289-297

[108] Carr G, Simmons NL, Sayer JA. Disruption of clc-5 leads to a redistribution of annexin A2 and promotes calcium crystal agglomeration in collecting duct epithelial cells. Cellular and Molecular Life Sciences. 2006;**3**:367-377

[109] Sorokina EA, Kleinman JG. Cloning and preliminary characterization of a calcium-binding protein closely related to nucleolin on the apical surface of inner medullary collecting duct cells. Journal of Biological Chemistry. 1999;**39**:27491-27496

[110] Verkoelen CF. Crystal retention in renal stone disease: A crucial role for the glycosaminoglycan hyaluronan? Journal of the American Society of Nephrology. 2006;**17**:1673-1687

[111] Khan A, Wang W, Khan SR. Calcium oxalate nephrolithiasis and expression of matrix GLA protein in the kidneys. World Journal of Urology. 2014;**32**:123-130

[112] Lieske JC, Leonard R, Toback FG. Adhesion of calcium oxalate monohydrate crystals to renal epithelial cells is inhibited by specific anions. American Journal of Physiology. 1995;**268**:F604-F612

[113] Lieske JC, Walsh-Reitz MM, Toback FG. Calcium oxalate monohydrate crystals are endocytosed by renal epithelial cells and induce proliferation. American Journal of Physiology. 1992;**262**:F622-F630

[114] Umekawa T, Chegini N, Khan SR. Oxalate ions and calcium oxalate crystals stimulate MCP-1 expression by renal epithelial cells. Kidney International. 2002;**61**:105-112

[115] Aihara K, Byer KJ, Khan SR. Calcium phosphate-induced renal epithelial injury and stone formation: Involvement of reactive oxygen species. Kidney International. 2003;**4**:1283-1291

[116] Thamilselvan S, Khan SR, Menon M. Oxalate and calcium oxalate mediated free radical toxicity in renal epithelial cells: Effect of antioxidants. Urological Research. 2003;**1**:3-9

[117] Umekawa T, Chegini N, Khan SR. Increased expression of monocyte chemoattractant protein-1 (MCP-1) by renal epithelial cells in culture on exposure to calcium oxalate, phosphate and uric acid crystals. Nephrology Dialysis Transplantation. 2003;**4**:664-669

[118] Verkoelen CF, van der Boom BG, Houtsmuller AB, Schroder FH, Romijn JC. Increased calcium oxalate monohydrate crystal binding to injured renal tubular epithelial cells in culture. American Journal of Physiology. 1998;**274**:F958-F965

[119] Schepers MS, Van Ballegooijen ES, Bangma CH Verkoelen CF. Crystals cause acute necrotic cell death in renal proximal tubule cells, but not in collecting tubule cells. Kidney International. 2005;**68**:1543-1553

[120] Guo C, McMartin KE. The cytotoxicity of oxalate, metabolite of ethylene glycol, is due to calcium oxalate monohydrate formation. Toxicology. 2005;**208**:347-355

[121] Schepers MS, Van Ballegooijen ES, Bangma CH, Verkoelen CF. Oxalate is toxic to renal tubular cells only at supraphysiologic concentrations. Kidney International. 2005;**68**:1660-1669

[122] Marengo SR, Chen DH, Evan AP Sommer AJ, Stowe NT, Ferguson DG, Resnick MI, MacLennan GT. Continuous infusion of oxalate by minipumps induces calcium oxalate nephrocalcinosis. Urological Research. 2006;**34**:200-210

[123] Robertson, W. G. Potential role of fluctuations in the composition of renal tubular fluid through the nephron in the initiation of Randall's plugs and calcium oxalate crystalluria in a computer model of renal function. Urolithiasis. 2015;**43**:93-107

[124] Marangella M. Bagnis C, Bruno M, Vitale C, Petrarulo M, Ramello A. Crystallization inhibitors in the pathophysiology and treatment of nephrolithiasis. Urologia Internationalis. 2004;**72**:6-10

[125] Kumar V, Lieske JC. Protein regulation of intrarenal crystallization. Current Opinion in Nephrology and Hypertension. 2006;**15**:374-380

[126] Gill WB, Jones KW, Ruggiero KJ. Protective effects of heparin and other sulfated glycosaminoglycans on crystal adhesion to injured urothelium. Journal of Urology. 1982;**127**:152-154

[127] Gambaro G, Trinchieri A. Recent advances in managing and understanding nephrolithiasis/nephrocalcinosis. F1000Res. 2016;**5**:1-8

[128] Kok DJ, Papapoulos SE, Blomen LJMJ, Bijvoet OLM. Modulation of calcium oxalate monohydrate crystallization kinetics in vitro. Kidney International. 1988;**34**:346-350

[129] Fleisch H. Inhibitors and promoters of stone formation. Kidney International. 1978;**13**:361-371;Grases F, Conte A. Urolithiasis, inhibitors and promoters. Urological Research. 1992;**20**:86-88

[130] Ryall RL, Harnett RM, Marshall VR. The effect of urine, pyrophosphate, citrate, magnesium and glycosaminoglycans on the growth and aggregation of calcium oxalate crystals in vitro. Clinica Chimica Acta. 1981;**112**:349-356

[131] Worcester EM, Blumenthal SS, Beshensky AM, Lewand DL. The calcium oxalate crystal growth inhibitor protein produced by mouse kidney cortical cells in culture is osteopontin. Journal of Bone and Mineral Research. 1992;**7**:1029-1036

[132] Worcester EM, Kleinman JG, Beshensky AM. Osteopontin production by cultured kidney cells. Annals of the New York Academy of Sciences. 1995;**760**:266-278

[133] Wesson JA, Ganne V, Beshensky AM, Kleinman JG. Regulation by macromolecules of calcium oxalate crystal aggregation in stone formers. Urological Research. 2005;**33**:206-212

[134] Viswanathan P, Rimer JD, Kolbach AM, Ward MD, Kleinman JG, Wesson JA. Calcium oxalate monohydrate aggregation induced by aggregation of desialylated Tamm-Horsfall protein. Urological Research. 2011;**39**:269-282

[135] Mo L, Huang HY, Zhu XH, Shapiro E, Hasty DL, Wu XR. Tamm-Horsfall protein is a critical renal defense factor protecting against calcium oxalate crystal formation. Kidney International. 2004;**66**:1159-1166

[136] Lien YH, Lai LW. Liposome-mediated gene transfer into the tubules. Experimental Nephrology. 1997;**5**:132-136

[137] Kumar V, Farell G, Lieske JC. Whole urinary proteins coat calcium oxalate monohydrate crystals to greatly decrease their adhesion to renal cells. Journal of Urology. 2003;**170**:221-225

[138] Verhulst A, Asselman M, De Naeyer S Vervaet BA, Mengel M, Gwinner W, D'Haese PC, Verkoelen CF, De Broe ME. Preconditioning of the distal tubular epithelium of the human kidney precedes nephrocalcinosis. Kidney International. 2005;**68**:1643-1647

[139] Pinheiro HS, Camara NO, Osaki KS, De Moura LA, Pacheco-Silva A. Early presence of calcium oxalate deposition in kidney graft biopsies is associated with poor long-term graft survival. American Journal of Transplantation. 2005;**5**:323-329

[140] Abitbol CL, Bauer CR, Montane B, Chandar J, Duara S, Zilleruelo G. Long-term follow-up of extremely low birth weight infants with neonatal renal failure. Pediatric Nephrology. 2003;**18**:887-893

[141] Lieske JC, Swift H, Martin T, Patterson B, Toback FG. Renal epithelial cells rapidly bind and internalize calcium oxalate monohydrate crystals. Proceedings of the National Academy of Sciences of the United States of America. 1994;**91**:6987-6991

[142] Lieske JC, Norris R, Swift H, Toback FG. Adhesion, internalization and metabolism of calcium oxalate monohydrate crystals by renal epithelial cells. Kidney International. 1997;**52**:1291-1301

[143] Schepers MS, Duim RA, Asselman M, Romijn JC, Schröder FH, Verkoelen CF. Internalization of calcium oxalate crystals by renal tubular cells: A nephron segment-specific process? Kidney International. 2003;**64**:493-500

[144] Chandhoke PS, Fan J. Transport of oxalate across the rabbit papillary surface epithelium. Journal of Urology. 2000;**164**:1724-1728

[145] Grover PK, Thurgood LA, Fleming DE, van Bronswijk W, Wang T, Ryall RL. Intracrystalline urinary proteins facilitate degradation and dissolution of calcium oxalate crystals in cultured renal cells. American Journal of Physiology Renal Physiology. 2008;**294**:F355-F361

[146] Chiangjong W, Thongboonkerd V. Calcium oxalate crystals increased enolase-1 secretion from renal tubular cells that subsequently enhanced crystal and monocyte invasion through renal interstitium. Science Reports. 2016;**6**:24064

[147] Fong-Ngern K, Peerapen P, Sinchaikul S, Chen ST, Thongboonkerd V. Large-scale identification of calcium oxalate monohydrate crystal-binding proteins on apical membrane of distal renal tubular epithelial cells. Journal of Proteome Research. 2011;**10**:4463-4477

[148] de Water R, Noordermeer C, van der Kwast TH, Nizze H, Boevé ER, Kok DJ, Schröder FH. Calcium oxalate nephrolithiasis: Effect of renal crystal deposition on the cellular composition of the renal interstitium. American Journal of Kidney Diseases. 1999;**33**:761-771

[149] De Bruijn WC, Boeve ER, van Run PR, van Miert PP, de Water R, Romijn JC, Verkoelen CF, Cao LC, Schrder FH. Etiology of calcium oxalate nephrolithiasis in rats. I. Can this be a model for human stone formation? Scanning Microscopy. 1995;**9**:103-114

[150] De Bruijn WC, Boeve ER, van Run PR,van Miert PP, Romijn JC, Verkoelen CF, Cao LC, Schröder FH. Etiology of experimental calcium oxalate monohydrate nephrolithiasis in rats. Scanning Microscopy. 1994;**8**:541-549

[151] Vervaet BA, Verhulst A, Dauwe SE, De Broe ME, D'Haese PC. An active renal crystal clearance mechanism in rat and man. Kidney International. 2008;**75**:41-51

[152] Markowitz GS, Nasr SH, Klein P, Anderson H, Stack JI, Alterman L, Price B, Radhakrishnan J, D'Agati VD. Renal failure due to acute nephrocalcinosis following oral sodium phosphate bowel cleansing. Human Pathology. 2004;**35**:675-684

[153] Low RK, Stoller ML. Endoscopic mapping of renal papillae for Randall's plaques in patients with urinary stone disease. Journal of Urology. 1997;**158**:2062-2064

[154] Bushinsky DA. Nephrolithiasis: Site of the initial solid phase. Journal of Clinical Investigation. 2003;**111**:602-605

[155] Khan SR, Glenton PA, Byer KJ. Modeling of hyperoxaluric calcium oxalate nephrolithiasis: Experimental induction of hyperoxaluria by hydroxy-L-proline. Kidney International. 2006;**70**:914-923.

[156] Peerapen P, Thongboonkerd V. Effects of calcium oxalate monohydrate crystals on expression and function of tight junction of renal tubular epithelial cells. Laboratory Investigation. 2011;**91**:97-105

[157] Peerapen P, Thongboonkerd V. p38 MAPK mediates calcium oxalate crystal-induced tight junction disruption in distal renal tubular epithelial cells. Scientific Reports. 2013;**3**:1041

[158] Asplin J, Mandel N, Coe F. Evidence for calcium phosphate supersaturation in the loop of Henle. American Journal of Physiology. 1996;**270**:F604-F613

[159] Khan SR, Canales BK. Ultrastructural investigation of crystal deposits in Npt2a knockout mice: Are they similar to human Randall's plaques? Journal of Urology. 2011;**186**:1107-1113

[160] Taylor ER, Stoller ML. Vascular theory of the formation of Randall plaques. Urolithiasis. 2014;**43**:41-45

[161] Randall A. The origin and growth of renal calculi. Annals of Surgery. 1937;**105**:1009-1027

[162] Randall A. Papillary pathology as a precursor of primary renal calculus. Journal of Urology. 1940;**44**:580-589

[163] Evan A, Lingeman J, Coe FL, Worcester E. Randall's plaque: Pathogenesis and role in calcium oxalate nephrolithiasis. Kidney International. 2006;**69**:1313-1318

[164] Miller NL, Gillen DL, Williams JC Jr, Evan AP, Bledsoe SB, Coe FL, Worcester EM, Matlaga BR, Munch LC, Lingeman JE. A formal test of the hypothesis that idiopathic calcium oxalate stones grow on Randall's plaque. BJU International. 2008;**103**:966-971

[165] Gambaro G, D'Angelo A, Fabris A, Tosetto E, Anglani F, Lupo A. Crystals, Randall's plaques and renal stones: Do bone and atherosclerosis teach us something? Journal of Nephrology. 2004;**17**:774-777

[166] Gambaro G, Fabris A, Abaterusso C, Cosaro A, Ceol M, Mezzabotta F, Torregrossa R, Tiralongo E, Del Prete D, D'Angelo A, Anglani F. Pathogenesis of nephrolithiasis: Recent insight from cell biology and renal pathology. Clinical Cases in Mineral and Bone Metabolism. 2008;**5**:107-109

[167] Gambaro G, Abaterusso C, Fabris A, Ruggera L, Zattoni F, Del Prete D, D'Angelo A, Anglani F. The origin of nephrocalcinosis, Randall's plaque and renal stones: A cell biology viewpoint. Archivio Italiano Di Urologia, Andrologia. 2009;**81**:166-170

[168] Khan SR, Gambaro G. Role of osteogenesis in the formation of Randall's plaques. Anatomical Record (Hoboken). 2016;**299**:5-7

[169] Iwano M, Plieth D, Danoff TM, Xue C, Okada H, Neilson EG. Evidence that fibroblasts derive from epithelium during tissue fibrosis. Journal of Clinical Investigation. 2002;**110**:341-350

[170] Rockey DC. The cell and molecular biology of hepatic fibrogenesis. Clinical and therapeutic implications. Clinical Liver Disease. 2000;**4**:319-355

[171] Boström K, Watson K, Horn S, Wortham C, Herman IM, Demer LL. Bone morphogenetic protein expression in human atherosclerotic lesions. Clinical Liver Disease. 1993;**91**:1800-1809

[172] Doherty MJ, Ashton BA, Walsh S, Beresford JN, Grant ME, Canfield AE. Vascular pericytes express osteogenic potential in vitro and in vivo. Journal of Bone and Mineral Research. 1998;**13**:828-838

[173] Cui L, Houston DA, Farquharson C, MacRae VE. Characterisation of matrix vesicles in skeletal and soft tissue mineralisation. Bone. 2016;**87**:147-158

[174] Boström K. Insights into the mechanism of vascular calcification. American Journal of Cardiology. 2001;**88**:20E-22E

[175] Shanahan CM, Cary NR, Salisbury JR, Proudfoot D, Weissberg PL, Edmonds ME. Medial localization of mineralization regulating proteins in association with Monckeberg's sclerosis: Evidence for smooth muscle cell-mediated vascular calcification. Circulation. 1999;**100**:2168-2176

[176] Proudfoot D, Skepper JN, Hegyi L, Bennett MR, Shanahan CM, Weissberg PL. Apoptosis regulates human vascular calcification in vitro: Evidence for initiation of vascular calcification by apoptotic bodies. Circulation Research. 2000;**87**:1055-1062

[177] Jono S, McKee MD, Murry CE, Shioi A, Nishizawa Y, Mori K, Morii H, Giachelli CM. Phosphate regulation of vascular smooth muscle cell calcification. Circulation Research. 2000;**87**:E10-E17

[178] Steitz SA, Speer MY, Curinga G, Yang HY, Haynes P, Aebersold R, Schinke T, Karsenty G, Giachelli CM. Smooth muscle cell phenotypic transition associated with calcification: Upregulation of Cbfa1 and downregulation of smooth muscle lineage markers. Circulation Research. 2001;**89**:1147-1154

[179] Doherty TM, Uzui H, Fitzpatrick LA, Tripathi PV, Dunstan CR, Asotra K, Rajavashisth TB. Rationale for the role of osteoclast-like cells in arterial calcification. FASEB Journal. 2002;**16**:577-582

[180] Proudfoot D, Davies JD, Skepper JN, Weissberg PL, Shanahan CM. Acetylated low-density lipoprotein stimulates human vascular smooth muscle cell calcification by promoting osteoblastic differentiation and inhibiting phagocytosis. Circulation. 2002;**106**:3044-3050

[181] Giachelli CM. Vascular calcification: In vitro evidence for the role of inorganic phosphate. Journal of the American Society of Nephrology. 2003;**14**:S300-S304

[182] Moe SM, Duan D, Doehle BP, O'Neill KD, Chen NX. Uremia induces the osteoblast differentiation factor Cbfa1 in human blood vessels. Kidney International. 2003;**63**:1003-1011

[183] Abedin M, Tintut Y, Demer LL. Vascular calcification: Mechanisms and clinical ramifications. Arteriosclerosis Thrombosis and Vascular Biology. 2004;**24**:1161-1170

[184] Giachelli CM. Vascular calcification mechanisms. Journal of the American Society of Nephrology. 2004;**15**:2959-2964

[185] Johnson RC, Leopold JA, Loscalzo J. Vascular calcification: Pathobiological mechanisms and clinical implication. Circulation Research. 2006;**99**:1044-1059

[186] Li X, Yang HY, Giachelli CM. BMP-2 promotes phosphate uptake, phenotypic modulation, and calcification of human vascular smooth muscle cells. Atherosclerosis. 2008;**199**:271-277

[187] Sage AP, Tintut Y, Demer LL. Regulatory mechanisms in vascular calcification. Nature Reviews Cardiology. 2010;**7**:528-536

[188] Yan J, Stringer SE, Hamilton A, Charlton-Menys V, Gotting C, Muller B, Aeschlimann D, Alexander MY. Decorin GAG synthesis and TGF-beta signaling mediate Ox-LDL-induced mineralization of human vascular smooth muscle cells. Arteriosclerosis Thrombosis and Vascular Biology. 2011;**31**:608-615

[189] Shroff R, Long DA, Shanahan C. Mechanistic insights into vascular calcification in CKD. Journal of the American Society of Nephrology. 2013;**24**:179-189

[190] Liao L, Zhou Q, Song Y, Wu W, Yu H, Wang S, Chen Y, Ye M, Lu L. Ceramide mediates Ox-LDL-induced human vascular smooth muscle cell calcification via p38 mitogen-activated protein kinase signaling. PLoS One. 2013;**8**:e82379. DOI: 10. 1371/journal. pone. 0082379

[191] Rong S, Zhao X, Jin X, Zhang Z, Chen L, Zhu Y, Yuan W. Vascular calcification in chronic kidney disease is induced by bone morphogenetic protein-2 via a mechanism involving the Wnt/β-catenin pathway. Cellular Physiology and Biochemistry. 2014;**34** (6):2049-2060

[192] Evrard S, Delanaye P, Kamel S, Cristol JP, Cavalier E. Vascular calcification: From pathophysiology to biomarkers. Clinica Chimica Acta. 2015;**438**:401-414

[193] Leopold JA. Vascular calcification: Mechanisms of vascular smooth muscle cell calcification. Trends in Cardiovascular Medicine. 2015;**25**(4):267-274. DOI: 10. 1016/j. tcm. 2014. 10. 021

[194] Canfield AE, Sutton AB, Hoyland JA, Schor AM. Association of thrombospondin-1 with osteogenic differentiation of retinal pericytes in vitro. Journal of Cell Science. 1996;**109(**Pt 2):343-353

[195] Golub EE. Biomineralization and matrix vesicles in biology and pathology. Seminars in Immunopathology. 2011;**33**:409-417

[196] Osman L, Yacoub MH, Latif N, Amrani M, Chester AH. Role of human valve interstitial cells in valve calcification and their response to atorvastatin. Circulation. 2006;**114**:I547-I552

[197] Demer LL, Tintut Y. Vascular calcification: Pathobiology of a multifaceted disease. Circulation. 2008;**117**:2938-2948

[198] Westendorf JJ, Kahler RA, Schroeder TM. Wnt signaling in osteoblasts and bone diseases. Gene. 2004;**341**:19-39

[199] Hill TP, Spater D, Taketo MM, Birchmeier W, Hartmann C. Canonical Wnt/beta-catenin signaling prevents osteoblasts from differentiating into chondrocytes. Developmental Cell. 2005;**8**:727-738

[200] Bodine PV, Komm BS. Wnt signaling and osteoblastogenesis. Reviews in Endocrine and Metabolic Disorders. 2006;**7**:33-39

[201] Martinez-Moreno JM, Munoz-Castaneda JR, Herencia C, Oca AM, Estepa JC, Canalejo R, Rodriguez-Ortiz ME, Perez-Martinez P, Aguilera-Tejero E, Canalejo A, Rodriguez M, Almaden Y. In vascular smooth muscle cells paricalcitol prevents phosphate-induced wnt/beta-catenin activation. American Journal of Physiology Renal Physiology. 2012;**303**:F1136-F1144

[202] Lee HL, Woo KM, Ryoo HM, Baek JH. Tumor necrosis factor-alpha increases alkaline phosphatase expression in vascular smooth muscle cells via MSX2 induction. Biochemical and Biophysical Research Communications. 2010;**391**:1087-1092

[203] Mikhaylova L, Malmquist J, Nurminskaya M. Regulation of in vitro vascular calcification by BMP4, VEGF and wnt3a. Calcified Tissue International. 2007;**81**:372-381

[204] Shao JS, Cheng SL, Pingsterhaus JM, Charlton-Kachigian N, Loewy AP, Towler DA. Msx2 promotes cardiovascular calcification by activating paracrine wnt signals. Journal of Clinical Investigation. 2005;**115**:1210-1220

[205] Mizobuchi M, Towler D, Slatopolsky E. Vascular calcification: The killer of patients with chronic kidney disease. Journal of the American Society of Nephrology. 2009;**20**:1453-1464

[206] Bostrom KI, Rajamannan NM, Towler DA. The regulation of valvular and vascular sclerosis by osteogenic morphogens. Circulation Research. 2011;**109**:564-577

[207] Gaur T, Lengner CJ, Hovhannisyan H, Bhat RA, Bodine PV, Komm BS, Javed A, van Wijnen AJ, Stein JL, Stein GS, Lian JB. Canonical wnt signaling promotes osteogenesis by directly stimulating runx2 gene expression. The Journal of Biological Chemistry. 2005;**280**:33132-33140

[208] Lian JB, Stein GS, Javed A, van Wijnen AJ, Stein JL, Montecino M, Hassan MQ, Gaur T, Lengner CJ, Young DW. Networks and hubs for the transcriptional control of osteoblastogenesis. Reviews in Endocrine and Metabolic Disorders. 2006;**7**:1-16

[209] Nakashima K, Zhou X, Kunkel G, Zhang Z, Deng JM, Behringer RR, de Crombrugghe B. The novel zinc finger-containing transcription factor osterix is required for osteoblast differentiation and bone formation. Cell. 2002;**108**:17-29

[210] Zhu F, Friedman MS, Luo W, Woolf P, Hankenson KD. The transcription factor osterix (SP7) regulates BMP6-induced human osteoblast differentiation. Journal of Cellular Physiology. 2012;**227**:2677-2685

[211] Giachelli CM, Bae N, Almeida M, Denhardt DT, Alpers CE, Schwartz SM. Osteopontin is elevated during neo-intima formation in rat arteries and is a novel component of human atherosclerotic plaques. Journal of Clinical Investigation. 1993;**92**:1686-1696

[212] Ikeda T, Shirasawa T, Esaki Y, Yoshiki S, Hirokawa K. Osteopontin mRNA is expressed by smooth muscle-derived foam cells in human atherosclerotic lesions of the aorta. Journal of Clinical Investigation. 1993;**92**:2814-2820

[213] Hirota S, Imakita M, Kohri K, Ito A, Morii E, Adachi S, Kim HM, Kitamura Y, Yutani C, Nomura S. Expression of osteopontin messenger RNA by macrophages in atherosclerotic plaques. A possible association with calcification. American Journal of Pathology. 1993;**143**:1003-1008

[214] Shanahan CM, Cary NR, Metcalfe JC, Weissberg PL. High expression of genes for calcification-regulating proteins in human atherosclerotic plaques. Journal of Clinical Investigation. 1994;**93**:2393-2402

[215] Dhore CR, Cleutjens JP, Lutgens E, Cleutjens KB, Geusens PP, Kitslaar PJ, Tordoir JH, Spronk HM, Vermeer C, Daemen MJ. Differential expression of bone matrix regulatory proteins in human atherosclerotic plaques. Arteriosclerosis Thrombosis and Vascular Biology. 2001;**21**:1998-2003

[216] Bennett BJ, Scatena M, Kirk EA, Rattazzi M, Varon RM, Averill M, Schwartz SM, Giachelli CM, Rosenfeld ME. Osteoprotegerin inactivation accelerates advanced atherosclerotic lesion progression and calcification in older ApoE-/- mice. Arteriosclerosis Thrombosis and Vascular Biology. 2006;**26**:2117-2124

[217] Shanahan CM, Crouthamel MH, Kapustin A, Giachelli CM. Arterial calcification in chronic kidney disease: Key roles for calcium and phosphate. Circulation Research. 2011;**109**:697-711

[218] Jahnen-Dechent W, Heiss A, Schafer C, Ketteler M. Fetuin-A regulation of calcified matrix metabolism. Circulation Research. 2011;**108**:1494-1509

[219] Heiss A, DuChesne A, Denecke B, Grotzinger J, Yamamoto K, Renne T, Jahnen-Dechent W. Structural basis of calcification inhibition by alpha 2-HS glycoprotein/fetuin-A. Formation of colloidal calciprotein particles. The Journal of Biological Chemistry. 2003;**278**:13333-13341

[220] Pal SN, Golledge J. Osteoprogenitors in vascular calcification: A circulating cell theory. Journal of Atherosclerosis and Thrombosis. 2011;**18**:551-559

[221] Tang Z, Wang A, Yuan F, Yan Z, Liu B, Chu JS, Helms JA, Li S. Differentiation of multipotent vascular stem cells contributes to vascular diseases. Nature Communications. 2012;**3**:875

[222] Kendrick J, Chonchol M. The role of phosphorus in the development and progression of vascular calcification. American Journal of Kidney Diseases. 2011;**58**:826-834

[223] Villa-Bellosta R, Bogaert YE, Levi M, Sorribas V. Characterization of phosphate transport in rat vascular smooth muscle cells: Implications for vascular calcification. Arteriosclerosis Thrombosis and Vascular Biology. 2007;**27**:1030-1036

[224] Villa-Bellosta R. Vascular calcification revisited: A new perspective for phosphate transport. Current Cardiology Reviews. 2015;**11**:341-351

[225] Li X, Yang HY, Giachelli CM. Role of the sodium-dependent phosphate cotransporter, Pit-1, in vascular smooth muscle cell calcification. Circulation Research. 2006;**98**:905-912

[226] Kapustin AN, Davies JD, Reynolds JL, McNair R, Jones GT, Sidibe A, Schurgers LJ, Skepper JN, Proudfoot D, Mayr M, Shanahan CM. Calcium regulates key components of vascular smooth muscle cell-derived matrix vesicles to enhance mineralization. Circulation Research. 2011;**109**:e1-e12

[227] Sutra T, Morena M, Bargnoux AS, Caporiccio B, Canaud B, Cristol JP. Superoxide production: A procalcifying cell signalling event in osteoblastic differentiation of vascular smooth muscle cells exposed to calcification media. Free Radical Biology & Medicine. 2008;**42**:789-797

[228] Byon CH, Javed A, Dai Q, Kappes JC, Clemens TL, Darley-Usmar VM, McDonald JM, Chen Y. Oxidative stress induces vascular calcification through modulation of the osteogenic transcription factor Runx2 by AKT signaling. The Journal of Biological Chemistry. 2008;**283**:15319-15327

[229] Parhami F, Morrow AD, Balucan J, Leitinger N, Watson AD, Tintut Y, Berliner JA, Demer LL. Lipid oxidation products have opposite effects on calcifying vascular cell and bone cell differentiation. A possible explanation for the paradox of arterial calcification in osteoporotic patients. Arteriosclerosis Thrombosis and Vascular Biology. 1997;**17**:680-687

[230] Tintut Y, Patel J, Parhami F, Demer LL. Tumor necrosis factor-alpha promotes in vitro calcification of vascular cells via the cAMP pathway. Circulation. 2000;**102**:2636-2642

[231] Tintut Y, Patel J, Territo M, Saini T, Parhami F, Demer LL. Monocyte/macrophage regulation of vascular calcification in vitro. Circulation. 2002;**105**:650-655

[232] Aikawa E, Nahrendorf M, Figueiredo JL, Swirski FK, Shtatland T, Kohler RH, Jaffer FA, Aikawa M, Weissleder R. Osteogenesis associates with inflammation in early-stage atherosclerosis evaluated by molecular imaging in vivo. Circulation. 2007;**116**:2841-2850

[233] Shanahan CM. Inflammation ushers in calcification: A cycle of damage and protection? Circulation. 2007;**116**:2782-2785

[234] Smith ER, Ford ML, Tomlinson LA, Rajkumar C, McMahon LP, Holt SG. Phosphorylated fetuin-A-containing calciprotein particles are associated with aortic stiffness and a procalcific milieu in patients with pre-dialysis CKD. Nephrology Dialysis Transplantation. 2012;**27**:1957-1966

[235] Parhami F, Tintut Y, Ballard A, Fogelman AM, Demer LL. Leptin enhances the calcification of vascular cells: Artery wall as a target of leptin. Circulation Research. 2001;**88**:954-960

[236] Zeadin M, ButcherM, Werstuck G, KhanM, Yee CK, Shaughnessy SG. Effect of leptin on vascular calcification in apolipoprotein E-deficient mice. Arteriosclerosis Thrombosis and Vascular Biology. 2009;**29**:2069-2075

[237] Hill JA, Olson EN, Griendling KK, Kitsis RN, Stull JT, Sweeney HL, editors. Muscle: Fundamental Biology and Mechanisms of Disease. Elsevier Science & Technology Books. Oxford; 2012

[238] Jono S, Nishizawa Y, Shioi A, Morii H. 1,25-Dihydroxyvitamin D3 increases in vitro vascular calcification by modulating secretion of endogenous parathyroid hormone-related peptide. Circulation. 1998;**98**:1302-1306

[239] Shioi A, Mori K, Jono S, Wakikawa T, Hiura Y, Koyama H, Okuno Y, Nishizawa Y, Morii H. Mechanism of atherosclerotic calcification. Zeitschrift für Kardiologie. 2000;**89**(suppl 2): 75-79

[240] Patidar A, Singh DK, Winocour P, Farrington K, Baydoun AR. Human uraemic serum displays calcific potential in vitro that increases with advancing chronic kidney disease. Clinical Science (Lond). 2013;**125**:237-245

[241] Kurz P, Monier-Faugere MC, Bognar B, Werner E, Roth P, Vlachojannis J, Malluche HH. Evidence for abnormal calcium homeostasis in patients with adynamic bone disease. Kidney International. 1994;**46**:855-861

[242] Prie D, Torres PU, Friedlander G. A new axis of phosphate balance control: Fibroblast growth factor 23-Klotho. Journal of Nephrology. 2009;**5**:513-519

[243] Lim K, Lu TS, Molostvov G, Lee C, Lam FT, Zehnder D, Hsiao LL. Vascular Klotho deficiency potentiates the development of human artery calcification and mediates resistance to fibroblast growth factor 23. Circulation. 2012;**125**:2243-2255

[244] Norman PE, Powell JT. Vitamin D and cardiovascular disease. Circulation Research. 2014;**114**:379-393

[245] Stubbs JR, Liu S, Tang W, Zhou J, Wang Y, Yao X, Quarles LD. Role of hyperphosphatemia and 1,25-dihydroxyvitamin D in vascular calcification and mortality in fibroblastic growth factor 23 null mice. Journal of the American Society of Nephrology. 2007;**18**:2116-2124

[246] Norman PE, Powell JT. Vitamin D, shedding light on the development of disease in peripheral arteries. Arteriosclerosis Thrombosis and Vascular Biology. 2005;**25**:39-46

[247] Rachez C, Freedman LP. Mechanisms of gene regulation by vitamin D(3) receptor: A network of coactivator interactions. Gene. 2000;**246**:9-21

[248] Barsony J, Prufer K. Vitamin D receptor and retinoid X receptor interactions in motion. Vitamins and Hormones. 2002;**65**:345-376

[249] Lin R, Amizuka N, Sasaki T, Aarts MM, Ozawa H, Goltzman D, Henderson JE, White JH. 1Alpha,25-dihydroxyvitamin D3 promotes vascularization of the chondro-osseous junction by stimulating expression of vascular endothelial growth factor and matrix metalloproteinase 9. Journal of Bone and Mineral Research. 2002;**17**:1604-1612

[250] London GM, Guerin AP, Marchais SJ, Metivier F, Pannier B, Adda H. Arterial media calcification in end-stage renal disease: Impact on all-cause and cardiovascular mortality. Nephrology Dialysis Transplantation. 2003;**18**:1731-1740

[251] Mori K, Shioi A, Jono S, Nishizawa Y, Morii H. Dexamethasone enhances in vitro vascular calcification by promoting osteoblastic differentiation of vascular smooth muscle cells. Arteriosclerosis Thrombosis and Vascular Biology. 1999;**19**:2112-2118

[252] Kirton JP, Wilkinson FL, Canfield AE, Alexander MY. Dexamethasone downregulates calcification-inhibitor molecules and accelerates osteogenic differentiation of vascular pericytes: Implications for vascular calcification. Circulation Research. 2006;**98**:1264-1272

[253] Reynolds JL, Joannides AJ, Skepper JN, McNair R, Schurgers LJ, Proudfoot D, Jahnen-Dechent W, Weissberg PL, Shanahan CM. Human vascular smooth muscle cells undergo vesicle-mediated calcification in response to changes in extracellular calcium and phosphate concentrations: A potential mechanism for accelerated vascular calcification in ESRD. Journal of the American Society of Nephrology. 2004;**15**:2857-2867

[254] Kapustin AN, Shanahan CM. Calcium regulation of vascular smooth muscle cell derived matrix vesicles. Trends in Cardiovascular Medicine. 2012;**22**:133-137

[255] Demer LL, Tintut Y. Inflammatory, metabolic, and genetic mechanisms of vascular calcification. Arteriosclerosis Thrombosis and Vascular Biology. 2014;**34**:715-723

[256] Hofmann Bowman MA, McNally EM. Genetic pathways of vascular calcification. Trends in Cardiovascular Medicine. 2012;**22**:93-98

[257] Chen NX, O'Neill K, Chen X, Kiattisunthorn K, Gattone VH, Moe SM. Transglutaminase2 accelerates vascular calcification in chronic kidney disease. American Journal of Nephrology. 2013;**37**:191-198

[258] Kapustin A, Chatrou M, Kalra S, Drozdov I, Soong D, Furmanik M, Sanchis P, De Rosales RT, Alvarez-Hernandez D, Shroff R, Yin X, Muller K, Skepper JN, Mayr M, Reutelingsperger CP, Chester A, Bertazzo S, Schurgers LJ, Shanahan CM. Regulated exosome secretion by vascular smooth muscle cells mediates vascular calcification. Heart. 2014;**100**(suppl. 3):A93-A94

[259] Kim KM. Apoptosis and calcification. Scanning Microscopy. 1995;**9**:1137-1175

[260] Kockx MM, De Meyer GR, Muhring J, Jacob W, Bult H, Herman AG. Apoptosis and related proteins in different stages of human atherosclerotic plaques. Circulation 1998;**97**:2307-2315

[261] Giachelli CM, Speer MY, Li X, Rajachar RM, Yang H. Regulation of vascular calcification: Roles of phosphate and osteopontin. Circulation Research. 2005;**96**:717-722

[262] Hashimoto S, Ochs RL, Rosen F, Quach J, McCabe G, Solan J, Seegmiller JE, Terkeltaub R, Lotz M. Chondrocyte-derived apoptotic bodies and calcification of articular cartilage. Proceedings of the National Academy of Science of the United States. 1998;**95**:3094-3099

[263] Dai XY, Zhao MM, Cai Y, Guan QC, Zhao Y, Guan Y, Kong W, Zhu WG, Xu MJ, Wang X. Phosphate-induced autophagy counteracts vascular calcification by reducing matrix vesicle release. Kidney International. 2013;**83**:1042-1051

[264] Leopold JA. MicroRNAs regulate vascular medial calcification. Cells. 2014;**3**:963-980

[265] Kim JH, Kim K, Youn BU, Lee J, Kim I, Shin HI, Akiyama H, Choi Y, Kim N. Kruppel-like factor 4 attenuates osteoblast formation, function, and cross talk with osteoclasts. Journal of Cell Biology. 2014;**204**:1063-1074

[266] Goettsch C, Hutcheson JD, Aikawa E. MicroRNA in cardio-vascular calcification: Focus on targets and extracellular vesicle delivery mechanisms. Circulation Research. 2013;**112**:1073-1084

[267] Balderman JA, Lee HY, Mahoney CE, Handy DE, White K, Annis S, Lebeche D, Hajjar RJ, Loscalzo J, Leopold JA. Bone morphogenetic protein-2 decreases microRNA-30b and microRNA-30c to promote vascular smooth muscle cell calcification. Journal of the American Heart Association. 2012;**1**:e003905. DOI: 10. 1161/JAHA. 112. 003905

[268] Goettsch C, Rauner M, Pacyna N, Hempel U, Bornstein SR, Hofbauer LC. miR-125b regulates calcification of vascular smooth muscle cells. The American Journal of Pathology. 2011;**179**:1594-1600

[269] Kageyama S, Ohtawara Y, Fujita K, Watanabe T, Ushiyama T, Suzuki K, Naito Y, Kawabe K. Microlith formation in vitro by Madin Darby canine kidney (MDCK) cells. International Journal of Urology. 1996;**3**:23-26

[270] Naito Y, Ohtawara Y, Kageyama S, Nakano M, Ichiyama A, Fujita M, Suzuki K, Kawabe K, Kino I. Morphological analysis of renal cell culture models of calcium phosphate stone formation. Urological Research. 1997;**25**:59-65

[271] Senzaki H, Yasui T, Okada A, Ito Y, Tozawa K, Kohri K. Alendronate inhibits urinary calcium microlith formation in a three-dimensional culture model. Urological Research. 2004;**32**:223-228

[272] Chau H, El-Maadawy S, McKee MD, Tenenhouse HS. Renal calcification in mice homozygous for the disrupted type IIa Na/Pi cotransporter gene Npt2. Journal of Bone and Mineral Research. 2003;**18**:644-657

[273] Miyazawa K, Domini C, Moriyama MT, Suzuki K. Global analysis of expressed genes in renal epithelial cells exposed to calcium oxalate crystals. Urological Research. 2004;**32**:146

[274] Miyazawa K, Aihara K, Ikeda R, Moriyama MT, Suzuki K. cDNA macroarray analysis of genes in renal epithelial cells exposed to calcium oxalate crystals. Urological Research. 2009;**37**:27-33

[275] Azari F, Vali H, Guerquin-Kern J-L, Wue T-D, Croisy A, Sears SK, Tabrizian M, McKee MD. Intracellular precipitation of hydroxyapatite mineral and implications for pathologic calcification, Journal of Structural Biology. 2008;**162**:468-479

[276] Khan SR, Joshi S, Wang W. Dedifferentiation of renal epithelial cells into osteogenic cells and formation of Randall's plaque. Journal of the American Society of Nephrology. 2014b;**25**:101A

[277] Joshi S, Clapp WL, Wang W, Khan SR. Osteogenic changes in kidneys of hyperoxaluric rats. Biochimica et Biophysica Acta. 2015;**1852**:2000-2012

[278] Khan SR, Canales BK. Unified theory on the pathogenesis of Randall's plaques and plugs. Urolithiasis. 2015;**43**(Suppl 1):109-123

[279] Pallone TL, Silldorff EP. Pericyte regulation of renal medullary blood flow. Experimental Nephrology. 2001;**9**:165-170

Chapter 2

Metaphylaxis in Pediatric Urinary Stone Disease

Onur Kaygısız

Additional information is available at the end of the chapter

http://dx.doi.org/10.5772/intechopen.69982

Abstract

The high rate of recurrence of urinary stones after initial treatment makes metaphylaxis essential in children. Thorough assessment and planning prior to metaphylaxis enable accurate and effective treatment. Expected benefits and possible adverse conditions must be considered when deciding on dietary restrictions in growing children, as their bone development is ongoing. A diet that includes abundant hydration and avoids salt produces the optimal cost-benefit ratio. When dietary modification is not sufficient, medical treatment must be added.

Keywords: children, diet, food, and nutrition, kidney calculi, prevention, relapse

1. Introduction

The high rate of recurrence of urinary-stone disease indicates the necessity of metaphylaxis, especially in children. All lifestyle changes and medications for prevention of stone disease define the stone metaphylaxis. After stone treatment, even stone-free children showed a 25% recurrence rate during a three-year follow up [1]. In addition, after the urinary tract stone surgery, the rate of stone recurrence over five years has been observed to vary from 38 to 65% depending on the malformation of the urogenital system [2]. Children with metabolic disorders had a higher recurrence rate, so metabolic examination is essential to preventive treatment in children. In the pediatric age group, the most common metabolic disorders are hypercalciuria and hypocitraturia, with hypercalciuria more often found in the endemic areas and hypocitraturia in the nonendemic areas [3, 4]. Metaphylaxis has been found to reduce recurrence rates by about half, even in recurrent kidney stones [5].

Proper metaphylaxis must be preceded by a complete metabolic evaluation. In addition, identification of any anatomical abnormalities that may increase the risk of nephrolithiasis, a detailed dietary history, patient and family medical history, and a record of any medications used must be obtained [6].

The European Association of Urology (EAU) guidelines recommend metabolic assessment based on the type of the stones, which may be obtained spontaneously or after pediatric urolithiasis treatment [6]. However, it is not always possible to obtain stones with minimally invasive surgery, particularly in patients undergoing retrograde intrarenal surgery and shock wave lithotripsy (SWL). In this case, a general screening is required. The EAU's pediatric urology guidelines recommend biochemical testing, including serum urea, creatinine, electrolytes, phosphorus, alkaline phosphate, uric acid, total protein, and albumin. If hypercalcemia is identified, the level of parathormone should be measured [6]. The ratio of spot urine calcium to creatinine should be analyzed, including a urinalysis and urine culture. Calcium, phosphate, magnesium, oxalate, uric acid, citrate, cysteine, protein, and creatinine clearance must be measured in a 24-hour urine [6]. In some cases, the test can be customized based on the stone type.

Renal tubular acidosis (RTA) should be suspected in calcium stones with urine pH that repeatedly tests higher than 5.5 [7]. In such patients, blood-gas levels must be analyzed. A urine pH consistently testing lower than 6 may indicate an acidic arrest [7].

Any renal anomaly responsible for the stones should be treated if there is a treatable pathology, including ureteropelvic junction obstruction. The child's diet must be reviewed for risk factors, including anorexia, high salt intake, and excessive sugar intake. Metaphylaxis must take into consideration medically necessary diets, including ketogenic diets.

Urolithiasis of 1–2% is associated with use of some medications [8]. Detecting such risks in the medical history is important for proper treatment planning. Vitamins C and D, loop diuretics, carbonic anhydrase inhibitors, and laxatives affect the metabolism and may lead to stone formation. The mechanisms by which these drugs potentiate stone formation and the treatment approaches pertinent to them will be discussed later in this chapter [8]. Magnesium trisilicate, commonly used for gastroesophageal reflux, causes silica stones, and ciprofloxacin, sulfonamide, triamterene, indinavir, and ceftriaxone form stones [8–10] that are radiolucent or semiopaque [8]. Stones that are weakly opaque or nonopaque and for which analysis results cannot be obtained should be suspected as drug-induced calculi.

Excessive use of laxatives causes formation of ammonium acid urate stones. Low urine volume and the low pH associated with chronic diarrhea increase the ammonium in urine [8]. In addition, anorexia, which is usually a postpuberty disease, is a cause of urolithiasis, with 5% of anorexia patients forming kidney stones [11], which are usually calcium oxalate, but which may be ammonium urate [12, 13]. The latter being stones that develop in cases of decreased urinary output, increased urine ammonium with hypophosphaturia, and the hyperchloremic acidosis associated with diarrhea [14]. Anorexia and any other identified primary disease should be treated before metaphylaxis.

Loop diuretics are commonly used to treat pulmonary disorders in newborns and act on the Na^+-K^+-2Cl pump through the thick part of Henle's loop, inhibiting the reabsorption of magnesium and calcium with the reabsorption of sodium [15]. In infants, due to their low glomerular filtration rates and immature hepatic development, the half-life of drugs is 6–20-fold longer, the clearance is 1.2–1.4-fold lower, and volume distribution is 1.3–6-fold broader than in adults [15]. In addition, the half-life is further increased in premature infants, with a half-life that is 6 hours in term infants and as long as 67 hours in premature infants [16]. However, increased knowledge of the pharmacokinetics and complications of using loop diuretics in infants have decreased the incidence of stones associated with these drugs [17, 18].

2. Diet

2.1. Fluid intake

Metaphylaxis of urinary stones may primarily involve regulating fluid intake and diet. Although hydration has been shown to decrease stone recurrence, the effectiveness of nutrition is controversial [19]. Increased fluid intake increases urine volume and inhibits crystal supersaturation and crystallization. In children, the fluid intake required for adequate urinary output must be calculated over 1.5 l/m^{2}of body area [7]. Sweet-flavored liquids should be avoided, since fluid containing glucose and fructose increase excretion of calcium and oxalate [20]. In addition, fluid intake must be distributed over the entire day. Consequently, in metaphylaxis of stones, water intake is the approach that has the optimal cost-benefit ratio [21]. However, it is not possible to monitor the fluid intake of children in school, and children's compliance in hydration is poor in general [22]. Because the need for liquids varies with temperature and activity level, parents may be recommended to monitor hydration based on urine color and urine density, if possible. Urine densities that repeatedly measure higher than 1010 indicate inadequate fluid intake [22].

2.2. Nutrition

Eating fast foods and processed foods can potentiate increased salt intake, causing hypervolemia, which leads to decreased absorption of water and sodium through the proximal tubules. This, in turn, decreases the absorption of calcium by sodium in the proximal tubules, which increases the level of calcium in the urine. The concentration of sodium in the urine is in proportion to dietary salt intake. In turn, dietary salt intake is in direct proportion to the calcium excreted in the urine [23]. In a Western-type diet, salt intake is almost 9 g/day in adults, nearly 77% of which comes from processed foods [24]. In contrast, daily salt intake should be below 3 mEq/kg [25]. Therefore, children's consumption of fast foods should be limited to decrease dietary salt intake.

Only 10–20% of oxalate in the urine is associated with diet [26]. However, oxalate absorption through the bowels is related to dietary calcium intake [27], and restricting dietary calcium increases urinary excretion of oxalate. However, restricting salt decreases oxalate, and more significantly, the calcium excreted in the urine of those with calcium-oxalate stones [28].

Oxalate is the product of vitamin C metabolism and is excreted in urine [29]. Therefore, increased vitamin C intake may lead to hyperoxaluria. Children with hyperoxaluria should decrease consumption of high-oxalate foods [6]. In addition, oxalobacter formigenes, a probiotic, decreases urinary oxalate and is effective against hyperoxaluria [30].

Animal proteins increase the acid load, the excretion of calcium, and decrease the excretion of citrate [25]. In addition, purine metabolism increases uric acid [25], which increases the risk of calcium stones through epistaxis [31]. Despite all this, the protein restrictions recommended for adults are not suitable as part of stone metaphylaxis in children and adolescents, except in cases of definite indications [6].

Urinary excretion of citrate is affected by the system's acid-base balance. Although acidosis decreases renal excretion of citrate and increases its reabsorption, the opposite is true in alkalosis [32]. A Western-type diet that includes decreased consumption of fruits and vegetables and increased consumption of animal products causes metabolic acidosis, resulting in lower urine pH and hypocitraturia [33]. Hypokalemia also lowers urine pH, and low potassium intake decreases urine potassium and citrate in hypokalemia and increases urinary excretion of calcium [32, 34]. Systemic alkalization increases excretion of citrate, decreases excretion of calcium, and raises urine pH [35]. Oranges, lemons, limes, and some types of mandarins are natural sources of citrate [35]. Alkaline fruits, including melons, cause urinary alkalization [36]. Grapefruits increase excretion of both citrate and oxalate [37]. The lithogenic effects of grapefruit juice and apple juice are controversial [38, 39].

Metaphylaxis benefits may be provided by increasing hydration and citrus intake and decreasing intake of sodium, oxalate, animal protein, and fructose [32]. Cranberry juice is high in oxalate and, therefore, increases urinary calcium and oxalate and decreases uric acid concentration. However, cranberry juice acidifies the urine, resulting in increased formation of calcium-oxalate and urate stones but decreased formation of calcium-phosphate stones [40]. Since cranberry juice acidifies the urine, it may be useful for infection stones that have limited options for medical treatment [41].

A study of 42,859 adults showed that high coffee and tea intake decreased the risk of symptomatic stone formation [39]. A more recent study of 6033 adults suggested that coffee intake decreased urine oxalate and uric acid, increased urine calcium and potassium, and also decreased the supersaturation of calcium oxalate by increasing urine volume [42]. However, dietary intake of coffee and tea cannot be recommended for pediatric patients because of the lack of studies of these substances in children.

Potential renal acid load (PRAL) is used to calculate the acid load of foods in adults. However, renal net acid excretion (NAE), which is based on body area, is recommended for use in pediatric patients [43]. PRAL is calculated by the formula (mEq/d) = 0.49 × protein (g/d) + 0.037 × phosphorus (mg/d) − 0.021 × potassium (mg/d) − 0.026 × magnesium (mg/d) − 0.013 × calcium (mg/d) [43]. As the formula indicates, dietary protein and phosphorus have acidic effects, whereas potassium, magnesium, and calcium have alkaline effects.

3. Medical treatment

When dietary modification is insufficient for metaphylaxis of urinary stones, medical treatment must be a part of the plan.

3.1. Alkalizing agents

Urine alkalization is used to reduce recurrence of calcium oxalate, uric acid, and cysteine stones, and urine acidification is used to reduce recurrence of infection and calcium-phosphate stones. For urine alkalization, potassium citrate is chosen instead of sodium citrate because sodium causes hypercalciuria. Potassium citrate directly dissolves calcium-oxalate crystals [44]. Therefore, it has a protective effect, even on calcium-oxalate stones that have normal citrate levels. Potassium-citrate tablets are available in 5 and 10-mEq doses, and Shohl's citrate-containing solution, which contains 1 mEq of base per millimeter, may be used for infants and children who cannot use tablets.

For calcium-oxalate stones, the targeted urine pH is 6.5, because uric acid cannot dissolve urine pH lower than 5.5, as it needs more alkalinity to dissolve. In metaphylaxis for hyperuricosuria, the targeted pH is also 6.5; however, to dissolve small uric-acid stones, the targeted pH range is 7–7.2 [7]. The daily dose may include 1–3 mEq/kg, depending on the urine pH and the primary disease, and the dose may be as high as 5–8 mEq/kg for infants with distal RTA [45]. Ideally, three doses a day should be administered, and if only one dose is possible, it should be administered in the evening [46].

Alkalization with hydration and potassium citrate has effectively decreased the risk of stones in children who are on a ketogenic diet, but these children should be referred to pediatric neurology for treatment of their primary diseases before beginning alkalization treatment [47]. Because cysteine has poor solubility and precipitates when urine pH is between 5 and 7, in alkalization therapy, the targeted value of urine pH must be higher than 7.0 [6, 48]. Alkalization accompanied by hydration has effectively prevented the recurrence of cysteine stones [49, 50].

Acetazolamide, a carbonic anhydrase inhibitor, inhibits the reabsorption of sodium bicarbonate through the proximal tubules, thus raising urine pH and potentially resulting in metabolic acidosis with prolonged use. Including acetazolamide in citrate therapy at night significantly raises urine pH in patients with cysteine and uric-acid stones, but half of these patients discontinue the drug due to side effects [51]. In addition, high urine pH may lead to calcium-phosphate stones [52, 53].

3.2. Specific treatments according to metabolic disorder

3.2.1. Hypercalciuria

3.2.1.1. Thiazide-type diuretics

Thiazide-type diuretics are especially indicated for normokalemic idiopathic hypercalciuria, which may be either absorptive or renal. Absorptive hypercalciuria may develop as three types: type 1, with direct absorption of calcium through the gastrointestinal system; type 2, with absorption of calcium associated with 1.25 dihydroxyvitamin D; or type 3, with renal calcium and phosphate absorption [54, 55]. Resorptive hypercalciuria is caused by primary hyperparathyroidism and develops with increased bone demineralization [54].

Thiazide-type diuretics act on the distal tubules, in which 10% of the sodium chloride is reabsorbed by a thiazide-sensitive Na+/Cl carrier [56]. Salt restriction during the use of thiazide-type diuretics decreases its effectiveness. The side effects of using thiazides have been reported as hypokalemia, hyperglycemia, hypercalcemia, and renal injury [57, 58]. Hypokalemia occurs with high doses [56]. Hyperglycemia may develop when thiazides are used for hypertension, but it has not been observed when they are used for hypercalciuria indications [59]. There is little evidence of renal injury with prolonged use of low or medium doses [56]. Children who develop hypercalcemia during therapy must be examined for underlying, overlooked hyperparathyroidism [58]. The initial dose of hydrochlorothiazide is 1 mg/kg. High doses are associated with side effects [60]. Starting with a dose of 0.5 mg/kg and then titrating based on urine calcium levels enables both effective treatment and avoidance of side effects [61]. However, in cases where high doses of hydrochlorothiazide are necessary, including Dent disease, close follow-up for complications is required [60].

In the presence of calcium-phosphate stones, the possibility of hyperparathyroidism and RTA should be investigated [7]. In cases of high calcium and phosphate levels, it may have brushite-type crystallization in a narrow pH range (6.5–6.8) [7]. Carbonate apatite is crystallized at pH 6.8 or higher and may present with infection stones or calcium-oxalate stones [7]. Hydrochlorothiazide is also effective on brushite stones [7]. However, patients with these require urine acidification rather than urine alkalization. Cranberry juice may be recommended for pediatric patients, because L-methionine cannot be used for them [6, 7].

In idiopathic hypercalciuria, decreased bone density may affect future bone health [62]. Thiazide-derived diuretics support bone density, even in patients with restricted calcium [63]. Studies have suggested that hydrochlorothiazide is beneficial to bone density in children with hypercalciuria, but this effect has been reported as limited in older children who are developing osteopenia [64, 65]. Controlled studies with larger populations are needed, but early hydrochlorothiazide treatment appears to be favorable for bone growth.

3.2.2. Hyperoxaluria

3.2.2.1. Pyridoxine

Pyridoxine is used for primary hyperoxaluria (PH) type 1. PH has three types: type 1, a deficiency of alanine glyoxylate aminotransferase; type 2, a deficiency of D-glycerate dehydrogenase; and type 3, a deficiency of 4-hydroxy 2-oxoglutarate aldolase [66].

In PH, due to the enzyme deficiency, glyoxylate cannot be converted into glycine in cofactors of pyridoxine (vitamin B6). Therefore, excessive oxalate is produced by the lactate dehydrogenase enzyme in the liver. Type 1 is the severest form, and accounts for 80% of PH cases [67]. Children with PH type 1 may develop nephrocalcinosis and end-stage renal failure in addition to calcium-oxalate stones. In contrast, in PH type 3, no end-stage renal failure has been reported [68]. If PH is suspected in pediatric patients, it may be diagnosed using urinary oxalate values that have been corrected for body area. In children with PH, the normal oxalate level in 24-hour urine is 0.45 mmol/1.73 m^2/24-hour, and it is usually higher than 1 mmol/1.73 m^2/24-hour. If the oxalate level in 24-hour urine is higher than 0.7 mmol/1.73 m^2/24-hour in repeated tests, genetic examination should be performed after excluding causes for secondary hyperoxaluria. If it is not possible to diagnose with genetic examination despite high suspicion, enzyme activity should be analyzed in a liver biopsy [69]. In patients diagnosed with PH type 1, pyridoxine therapy should be prescribed in addition to hydration and citrate therapy. In type 1 PH, pyridoxine therapy is effective in 50% of patients and decreases the urinary-oxalate level by more than 30% [70]. New studies suggesting multiple effects of pyridoxine indicate promising ways to treat patients who have not benefited from existing treatments [71]. The initial pyridoxine dose is 5 mg/kg, and depending on the response, it can be titrated to 20 mg/kg. Although rare, sensorial neuropathy may develop with high doses [72].

Hyperoxaluria may also develop due to causes that include inflammatory bowel disease, short-bowel syndrome, ethylene-glycol intoxication, and excessive intake of vitamin C. In patients with secondary hyperoxaluria, dietary oxalate and salt restrictions and alkalization therapy should be begun, and in resistant patients, pyridoxine therapy should be used [6]. The initial dose of pyridoxine may be 2–5 mg/kg/day, and it can be titrated to 8–10 mg/kg/day.

3.2.3. Hyperuricosuria

3.2.3.1. Allopurinol

Hyperuricosuria occurs when uric acid is higher than 10 mg/kg in 24-hour urine [6]. Urinary excretion of uric acid is high in infants [26]. In acidic urine, solubility of uric acid is decreased. This is more apparent when pH is lower than 5.8 [6]. Hyperuricosuria not only causes uric-acid stones but also plays a role in forming calcium-oxalate stones through epistaxis [31]. If hydration and alkalization fail, allopurinol could be begun, particularly in children who have hyperuricosuria with hyperuricemia. Allopurinol inhibits the xanthine dehydrogenase enzyme, thereby decreasing the concentration of uric acid and increasing the concentration of xanthine in the urine [26]. The pediatric dose is 10 mg/kg [6]. Skin rashes may be seen, and very rarely, allopurinol hypersensitivity syndrome (AHS) may develop [73]. AHS is a fatal side effect that also includes a rash (Stevens-Johnson syndrome, toxic epidermal necrosis), eosinophilia, leukocytosis, hepatitis, fever, and renal failure [73]. This fatal complication has no specific treatment other than termination of treatment and support therapy [73]. Therefore, it is very important to educate patients and families about symptoms and to make an early diagnosis. To prevent such complications, it may be useful to begin with a low dose and increase it [73].

Hypoxanthine guanine phosphoribosyl transferase (HPRT) is a purine metabolism enzyme. HPRT deficiency, the severest form of which is Lesch-Nyhan syndrome, may occur with neurologic symptoms, mental retardation, and nephropathy, and in the early stages of life, kidney stones [74]. Deficiency of glucose-6-phosphate dehydrogenase leads to hyperuricemia, increasing the intracellular phosphoribosyl pyrophosphate in type 1 [75]. In both of these metabolic diseases, allopurinol therapy is indicated for hyperuricemia and hyperuricosuria. In addition to metabolic diseases, myeloproliferative diseases may also cause hyperuricosuria, and in children with hyperuricosuria who develop new stones and for whom hydration and alkalization are insufficient, allopurinol may be begun at 10 mg/kg [6].

Furthermore, deficiency of adenosine phosphoribosyl transferase (APRT), a purine metabolism enzyme, converts adenine into 8-hydroxyadenine and xanthine dehydrogenase enzyme into 2,8-dihydroxyadenine (DHA) [76]. Transfer of DHA into the urine is high, and its solubility is low, even in alkaline urine, so DHA stones form. Alkalization therapy is not useful in such cases, and therapy must consist of 5–10 mg/kg of allopurinol and sufficient hydration [77].

Xanthinuria has two types: type 1 develops with a deficiency of xanthine dehydrogenase enzyme and type 2 develops with a deficiency of aldehyde oxidase enzyme [78]. These two types are differentiated using an allopurinol test [78]. In addition, xanthinuria may develop after Lesh-Nyhan syndrome is treated using allopurinol [79]. Xanthinuria has no specific treatment but responds well to hydration, urine alkalization, and reduction of dietary purine [80].

3.2.4. Cystine stones

3.2.4.1. Drugs containing thiol

Cystinuria is a genetic disease in which reabsorption of cysteine and other dibasic amino acids, including ornithine, arginine, and lysine, through the proximal tubules is impaired [81]. Cystinuria has two genetic types: type 1, which is caused by the SLC3A1 gene on the 2nd chromosome and type 2, which is caused by the SLC7A9 gene on the 19th chromosome [82]. Cystinuria is more common in Eastern Mediterranean populations [83]. Cysteine higher than 50 mg/1.73 m^2 in 24-hour urine is considered as a diagnostic for cystinuria [26]. Where hydration and alkalization fail, use of thiol-containing drugs is recommended [6]. Thiol forms a disulfide complex, which is soluble with cysteine and prevents formation of stones. Thiol-containing drugs are more effective on alkaline urine, and a study has demonstrated that dissolution in urine incubated with cysteine was low for the first 60 minutes when the pH was 6, but it was optimal when the pH was 8 [84]. However, no difference was found between pH 7 and 8 after either 60 minutes or 48 hours [84]. This indicates the importance of alkalization even when using thiol-containing drugs. However, a high urine pH may lead to phosphate crystallization; therefore, pH 7–7.5 appears to be the most appropriate target.

D-penicillamine is a chelating agent that contains thiol and increases cysteine dissolution by as much as 50-fold [85]. D-penicillamine may cause bonemarrow suppression, proteinuria, skin eruptions on the neck and extremities, arthralgia, liver dysfunction, and febrile reaction [86]. Its use for metaphylaxis of cysteine stones is restricted by the fact that up to 86% of pediatric patients using it have developed side effects [87]. Although d-penicillamine use is not recommended in children, if it must be used, close follow-up for side effects is essential. In addition, to decrease side effects and increase tolerance, during the first week, the dose should be 5 mg/kg/day, and then it should be increased by 5 mg/kg/day, reaching 20 mg/kg/day at the end of four weeks [86]. Pyridoxine deficiency develops with long-term d- penicillamine therapy, so therapy should include pyridoxine [85].

Alfa mercaptopropionylglycine (AMG, thiopronin) has an effect similar to that of d-penicillamine but with fewer side effects [85]. The daily dose is 10–15 mg/kg [6]. The rate of treatment discontinuation is lower than that for d-penicillamine therapy [88]. Although thiopronin has fewer side effects than penicillamine, patients must be closely monitored for side effects, including fever, which often occurs during the first month, rash, bone marrow suppression, and nephrotic syndrome, which improves when the drug is ceased [89, 90]. One uncontrolled study suggested that giving a low dose or a dose every other day was effective and further decreased the side effects [91]. Use of thiopronin is recommended for pediatric patients when hydration and alkalization are not adequate to decrease cystinuria [6].

Adding **captopril** to cysteine makes the cysteine more than 200 times soluble in urine [86]. However, it lowers the concentration of captopril in the urine, making this treatment less effective than AMG or d-penicillamine [92, 93]. Case reports have shown that this treatment is effective in pediatric patients and has relatively few side effects, but some studies have also indicated the opposite [94–96]. The EAU's pediatric urology guidelines do not recommend the treatment, but it may be considered when AMG cannot be used because of side effects or in children with hypertension and proteinuria [6].

3.2.5. *Infection stones*

Infection stones are stones of struvite, carbonate apatite, or ammonium urate. Urease-positive bacteria increase urinary bicarbonate and ammonium, making urine basic [7]. Unlike acidic stones, ammonium-urate stones form in basic environments and are associated with urinary tract infections [7]. In the case of infection stones, the carbonate-apatite form of calcium phosphate crystalizes at pH 6.8 or higher [7].

In metaphylaxis of infection stones, the primary objective is complete elimination of the stones. If a renal anomaly is causing stasis, it should be treated. Use of urease inhibitors is controversial, even in adult patients, due to their high rate of complications, and L-methionine for urine acidification is not recommended in children [6, 7]. Intake of cranberry juice may be recommended for urine acidification in pediatric patients. Antibiotic therapy and prophylaxis may be begun if required, along with urinary-culture follow-up.

4. Conclusions

Frequent recurrence of urinary stones after initial treatment makes metaphylaxis crucial in children. Suitable metaphylaxis must be preceded by complete metabolic evaluation. Increasing fluid intake and optimizing the diet are the first steps in urinary-stone metaphylaxis. When these measures are not sufficient, medical treatment must be added. Most recommendations for metaphylaxis in children are based on studies involving adults, and, therefore, more studies involving children are called for.

Author details

Onur Kaygısız

Address all correspondence to: onurkygsz@yahoo.com

Faculty of Medicine, Department of Urology, Uludağ University, Bursa, Turkey

References

[1] Abhishek, Kumar J, Mandhani A, Srivastava A, Kapoor R, Ansari MS. Pediatric urolithiasis: Experience from a tertiary referral center. Journal of Pediatric Urology. 2013 Dec;**9**(6 Pt A):825-830. DOI: 10.1016/j.jpurol.2012.11.003

[2] Lao M, Kogan BA, White MD, Feustel PJ. High recurrence rate at 5-year followup in children after upper urinary tract stone surgery. Journal of Urology. 2014 Feb;**191**(2):440-444. DOI: 10.1016/j.juro.2013.09.021.)

[3] Elmacı AM, Ece A, Akın F. Pediatric urolithiasis: Metabolic risk factors and follow-up results in a Turkish region with endemic stone disease. Urolithiasis. 2014 Oct;**42**(5):421-426. DOI: 10.1007/s00240-014-0682-z

[4] Ertan P, Tekin G, Oger N, Alkan S, Horasan GD. Metabolic and demographic characteristics of children with urolithiasis in Western Turkey. Urological Research. 2011 Apr;**39**(2):105-110. DOI: 10.1007/s00240-010-0306-1

[5] Tekin A, Tekgul S, Atsu N, Bakkaloglu M, Kendi S. Oral potassium citrate treatment for idiopathic hypocitruria in children with calcium urolithiasis. Journal of Urology. 2002 Dec;**168**(6):2572-2574

[6] Tekgül S, Dogan HS, Erdem E, Hoebeke P, Kocvara R, Nijman R, et al. European Society Guidelines for Paediatric Urinary Stone Disease. Urology Limited Update March; EAU 2015. pp. 51-58

[7] Straub M, Strohmaier WL, Berg W, Beck B, Hoppe B, Laube N, et al. Diagnosis and metaphylaxis of stone disease. Consensus concept of the national working committee on stone disease for the upcoming german urolithiasis guideline. World Journal of Urology. 2005;**23**(5):309-323. Epub 2005 Nov 29. Review.)

[8] Daudon M, Jungers P. Drug-induced renal calculi: Epidemiology, prevention and management. Drugs. 2004;**64**(3):245-275

[9] Matlaga BR, Shah OD, Assimos DG. Drug-induced urinary calculi. Reviews in Urology. 2003 Fall;**5**(4):227-231

[10] Chutipongtanate S, Thongboonkerd V. Ceftriaxone crystallization and its potential role in kidney stone formation. Biochemical and Biophysical Research Communications. 2011 Mar 18;**406**(3):396-402. DOI: 10.1016/j.bbrc.2011.02.053

[11] Herzog W, Deter HC, Fiehn W, Petzold E. Medical findings and predictors of long-term physical outcome in anorexia nervosa: A prospective, 12-year follow-up study. Psychological Medicine. 1997 Mar;**27**(2):269-279

[12] Komori K, Arai H, Gotoh T, Imazu T, Honda M, Fujioka H. A case of ammonium urate urinary stones with anorexia nervosa. Hinyokika Kiyo. 2000 Sep;**46**(9):627-629. Review. Japanese

[13] Leaf DE, Bukberg PR, Goldfarb DS. Laxative abuse, eating disorders, and kidney stones: A case report and review of the literature. American Journal of Kidney Diseases. 2012 Aug;**60**(2):295-298. DOI: 10.1053/j.ajkd.2012.02.337

[14] Bouquegneau A, Dubois BE, Krzesinski JM, Delanaye P. Anorexia nervosa and the kidney. American Journal of Kidney Diseases. 2012 Aug;**60**(2):299-307. DOI: 10.1053/j.ajkd.2012.03.019

[15] Pacifici GM. Clinical pharmacology of furosemide in neonates: A review. Pharmaceuticals (Basel). 2013 Sep 5;**6**(9):1094-1129. DOI: 10.3390/ph6091094

[16] Young TE, Mangum B, Neofax A. Manual of Drugs used in Neonatal Care. Cardiovascular. 23rd ed. Montvale, NJ, USA: Thomson Reuters; 2010. pp. 248-249

[17] Hufnagle KG, Khan SN, Penn D, Cacciarelli A, Williams P. Renal calcifications: A complication of long-term furosemide therapy in preterm infants. Pediatrics. 1982 Sep;**70**(3):360-363

[18] Chang HY, Hsu CH, Tsai JD, Li ST, Hung HY, Kao HA, Chang JH, Chung HY, Wang HK. Renal calcification in very low birth weight infants. Pediatrics and Neonatology. 2011 Jun;**52**(3):145-149. DOI: 10.1016/j.pedneo.2011.03.004

[19] Fink HA, Akornor JW, Garimella PS, MacDonald R, Cutting A, Rutks IR, Monga M, Wilt TJ. Diet, fluid, or supplements for secondary prevention of nephrolithiasis: A systematic review and meta-analysis of randomized trials. European Urology. 2009 Jul;**56**(1):72-80. DOI: 10.1016/j.eururo.2009.03.031.Review

[20] Nguyen NU, Dumoulin G, Henriet MT, Regnard J. Increase in urinary calcium and oxalate after fructose infusion. Hormone and Metabolic Research. 1995 Mar;**27**(3):155-158

[21] Lotan Y, Buendia Jiménez I, Lenoir-Wijnkoop I, Daudon M, Molinier L, Tack I, Nuijten MJ. Increased water intake as a prevention strategy for recurrent urolithiasis: Major impact of compliance on cost-effectiveness. Journal of Urology. 2013 Mar;**189**(3):935-939. DOI: 10.1016/j.juro.2012.08.254

[22] Alon US, Zimmerman H, Alon M. Evaluation and treatment of pediatric idiopathic urolithiasis-revisited. Pediatric Nephrology. 2004 May;**19**(5):516-520

[23] Ticinesi A, Nouvenne A, Maalouf NM, Borghi L, Meschi T. Salt and nephrolithiasis. Nephrology Dialysis Transplantation. 2016 Jan;**31**(1):39-45. DOI: 10.1093/ndt/gfu243

[24] Mattes RD, Donnelly D. Relative contributions of dietary sodium sources. The Journal of the American College of Nutrition 1991;**10**:383-393

[25] Tasian GE, Copelovitch L. Evaluation and medical management of kidney stones in children. Journal of Urology. 2014 Nov;**192**(5):1329-1336. DOI: 10.1016/j.juro.2014.04.108

[26] Copelovitch L. Urolithiasis in children: Medical approach. Pediatric Clinics of North America. 2012 Aug;**59**(4):881-896. DOI: 10.1016/j.pcl.2012.05.009

[27] von Unruh GE, Voss S, Sauerbruch T, Hesse A. Dependence of oxalate absorption on the daily calcium intake. Journal of the American Society of Nephrology. 2004 Jun;**15**(6): 1567-1573

[28] Nouvenne A, Meschi T, Prati B, Guerra A, Allegri F, Vezzoli G, Soldati L, Gambaro G, Maggiore U, Borghi L. Effects of a low-salt diet on idiopathic hypercalciuria in calcium-oxalate stone formers: A 3-mo randomized controlled trial. Am J Clin Nutr. 2010 Mar;**91**(3):565-70. DOI: 10.3945/ajcn.2009.28614

[29] Curtin CO, King CG. The metabolism of ascorbic acid-1-C14 and oxalic acid-C14 in the rat. Journal of Biological Chemistry. 1955 Oct;**216**(2):539-548

[30] Jairath A, Parekh N, Otano N, Mishra S, Ganpule A, Sabnis R, Desai M. Oxalobacter formigenes: Opening the door to probiotic therapy for the treatment of hyperoxaluria. Scandinavian Journal of Urology. 2015 Feb 2:1-4

[31] Sarig S. The hyperuricosuric calcium oxalate stone former. Mineral and Electrolyte Metabolism. 1987;**13**(4):251-256

[32] Zuckerman JM, Assimos DG. Hypocitraturia: Pathophysiology and medical management. Reviews in Urology. 2009 Summer;**11**(3):134-144

[33] Adeva MM, Souto G. Diet-induced metabolic acidosis. Clinical Nutrition. 2011 Aug;**30**(4):416-421. DOI: 10.1016/j.clnu.2011.03.008

[34] Domrongkitchaiporn S, Stitchantrakul W, Kochakarn W. Causes of hypocitraturia in recurrent calcium stone formers: Focusing on urinary potassium excretion. American Journal of Kidney Diseases. 2006 Oct;**48**(4):546-554

[35] Heilberg IP, Goldfarb DS. Optimum nutrition for kidney stone disease. Advances in Chronic Kidney Disease. 2013 Mar;**20**(2):165-174. DOI: 10.1053/j.ackd.2012.12.001. Review

[36] Baia Lda C, Baxmann AC, Moreira SR, Holmes RP, Heilberg IP. Noncitrus alkaline fruit: A dietary alternative for the treatment of hypocitraturic stone formers. Journal of Endourology. 2012 Sep;**26**(9):1221-1226. DOI: 10.1089/end.2012.0092

[37] Goldfarb DS, Asplin JR. Effect of grapefruit juice on urinary lithogenicity. Journal of Urology. 2001 Jul;**166**(1):263-267

[38] Curhan GC, Willett WC, Rimm EB, Spiegelman D, Stampfer MJ. Prospective study of beverage use and the risk of kidney stones. American Journal of Epidemiology. 1996 Feb 1;**143**(3):240-247

[39] Hönow R, Laube N, Schneider A, Kessler T, Hesse A. Influence of grapefruit-, orange- and apple-juice consumption on urinary variables and risk of crystallization. British Journal of Nutrition. 2003 Aug;**90**(2):295-300

[40] Gettman MT, Ogan K, Brinkley LJ, Adams-Huet B, Pak CY, Pearle MS. Effect of cranberry juice consumption on urinary stone risk factors. Journal of Urology. 2005 Aug;**174**(2):590-594

[41] Kessler T, Jansen B, Hesse A. Effect of blackcurrant-, cranberry- and plum juice consumption on risk factors associated with kidney stone formation. European Journal of Clinical Nutrition. 2002 Oct;**56**(10):1020-1023

[42] Ferraro PM, Taylor EN, Gambaro G, Curhan GC. Caffeine intake and the risk of kidney stones. The American Journal of Clinical Nutrition. 2014 Dec;**100**(6):1596-1603. DOI: 10.3945/ajcn.114.089987

[43] Remer T, Dimitriou T, Manz F. Dietary potential renal acid load and renal net acid excretion in healthy, free-living children and adolescents. The American Journal of Clinical Nutrition. 2003 May;**77**(5):1255-1260

[44] Shang YF, Xu M, Zhang GN, Ouyang JM. Concave urinary crystallines: Direct evidence of calcium oxalate crystals dissolution by citrate in vivo. Bioinorganic Chemistry and Applications. 2013;**2013**:637617. DOI: 10.1155/2013/637617

[45] Batlle D, Haque SK. Genetic causes and mechanisms of distal renal tubular acidosis. Nephrology Dialysis Transplantation. 2012 Oct;**27**(10):3691-3704. DOI: 10.1093/ndt/gfs442. Review

[46] Berg C, Larsson L, Tiselius HG. Effects of different doses of alkaline citrate on urine composition and crystallization of calcium oxalate. Urological Research. 1990;**18**(1):13-16

[47] Sampath A, Kossoff EH, Furth SL, Pyzik PL, Vining EP. Kidney stones and the ketogenic diet: Risk factors and prevention. Journal of Child Neurology. 2007 Apr;**22**(4):375-378

[48] Claes DJ, Jackson E. Cystinuria: Mechanisms and management. Pediatric Nephrology. 2012 Nov;**27**(11):2031-2038. DOI: 10.1007/s00467-011-2092-6. Epub 2012 Jan 27. Review

[49] Izol V, Aridogan IA, Karsli O, Deger M, Satar N. The effect of prophylactic treatment with Shohl's solution in children with cystinuria. Journal of Pediatric Urology. 2013 Dec;**9**(6 Pt B):1218-1222. DOI: 10.1016/j.jpurol.2013.05.017

[50] Kizilöz H, Kaygisiz O, Çanakli F, Bilen CY, Erkan I, Tekgül S. The Effect of cystine level and urinary PH on the recurrence of cystine stones. Journal of Pediatric Urology. 2009 Apr;**5**(supp 1):s33

[51] Sterrett SP, Penniston KL, Wolf Jr JS, Nakada SY. Acetazolamide is an effective adjunct for urinary alkalization in patients with uric acid and cystine stone formation recalcitrant to potassium citrate. Urology. 2008 Aug;**72**(2):278-281. DOI: 10.1016/j.urology.2008.04.003

[52] Grases F, Zelenková M, Söhnel O. Structure and formation mechanism of calcium phosphate concretions formed in simulated body fluid. Urolithiasis. 2014 Feb;**42**(1):9-16. DOI: 10.1007/s00240-013-0611-6

[53] Kamel KS, Shafiee MA, Cheema-Dhadli S, Halperin ML. Studies to identify the basis for an alkaline urine pH in patients with calcium hydrogen phosphate kidney stones. Nephrology Dialysis Transplantation. 2007 Feb;**22**(2):424-431

[54] Bataille P, Fardellone P, Ghazali A, Cayrolle G, Hottelart C, Achard JM, Fournier A. Pathophysiology and treatment of idiopathic hypercalciuria. Current Opinion in Rheumatology. 1998 Jul;**10**(4):373-388

[55] Srivastava T, Schwaderer A. Diagnosis and management of hypercalciuria in children. Current Opinion in Pediatrics. 2009 Apr;**21**(2):214-219. DOI: 10.1097/MOP.0b013e3283223db7. Review

[56] Ellison DH, Loffing J. Thiazide effects and adverse effects: Insights from molecular genetics. Hypertension. 2009 Aug;**54**(2):196-202. DOI: 10.1161/HYPERTENSIONAHA.109.129171

[57] Frenkel NJ, Vogt L, De Rooij SE, Trimpert C, Levi MM, Deen PM, van den Born BJ. Thiazide-induced hyponatraemia is associated with increased water intake and impaired urea-mediated water excretion at low plasma antidiuretic hormone and urine aquaporin-2. Journal of Hypertension. 2015 Mar;**33**(3):627-633. DOI: 10.1097/HJH.0000000000000423

[58] Wermers RA, Kearns AE, Jenkins GD, Melton LJ. Incidence and clinical spectrum of thiazide-associated hypercalcemia. 3rd. American Journal of Medicine. 2007 Oct;**120**(10):911.e9-15. Epub 2007 Apr 16

[59] Singh P, Knoedler JJ, Krambeck AE, Lieske JC, Bergstralh EJ, Rule AD. Thiazide diuretic prophylaxis for kidney stones and the risk of diabetes mellitus. Journal of Urology. 2014 Dec;**192**(6):1700-1704. DOI: 10.1016/j.juro.2014.06.078

[60] Blanchard A, Vargas-Poussou R, Peyrard S, Mogenet A, Baudouin V, Boudailliez B, Charbit M, Deschesnes G, Ezzhair N, Loirat C, Macher MA, Niaudet P, Azizi M. Effect of hydrochlorothiazide on urinary calcium excretion in dent disease: An uncontrolled trial. American Journal of Kidney Diseases. 2008 Dec;**52**(6):1084-1095. DOI: 10.1053/j.ajkd.2008.08.021

[61] Choi JN, Lee JS, Shin JI. Low-dose thiazide diuretics in children with idiopathic renal hypercalciuria. Acta Paediatrica. 2011 Aug;**100**(8):e71-e74. DOI: 10.1111/j.1651-2227.2011.02191.x

[62] Zerwekh JE. Bone disease and hypercalciuria in children. Pediatric Nephrology. 2010 Mar;**25**(3):395-401. DOI: 10.1007/s00467-009-1338-z

[63] Pak CY, Heller HJ, Pearle MS, Odvina CV, Poindexter JR, Peterson RD. Prevention of stone formation and bone loss in absorptive hypercalciuria by combined dietary and pharmacological interventions. Journal of Urology. 2003 Feb;**169**(2):465-469

[64] Moreira Guimarães Penido MG, de Sousa Tavares M, Campos Linhares M, Silva Barbosa AC, Cunha M. Longitudinal study of bone mineral density in children with idiopathic hypercalciuria. Pediatric Nephrology. 2012 Jan;**27**(1):123-130. DOI: 10.1007/s00467-011-1952-4

[65] García-Nieto V, Monge-Zamorano M, González-García M, Luis-Yanes MI. Effect of thiazides on bone mineral density in children with idiopathic hypercalciuria. Pediatric Nephrology. 2012 Feb;**27**(2):261-268. DOI: 10.1007/s00467-011-1987-96

[66] Lorenzo V, Torres A, Salido E. Primary hyperoxaluria. Nefrologia. 2014 May 21;**34**(3):398-412. DOI: 10.3265/Nefrologia.pre2014.Jan.12335.[Article in English, Spanish]

[67] Fargue S. Factors influencing clinical outcome in patients with primary hyperoxaluria type 1. Kidney International. 2014 Dec;**86**(6):1074-1076. DOI: 10.1038/ki.2014.280

[68] Cochat P, Rumsby G. Primary hyperoxaluria. The New England journal of Medicine. 2013 Aug;**369**(7):649-658. DOI: 10.1056/NEJMra1301564. Review

[69] Milliner DS. The primary hyperoxalurias: An algorithm for diagnosis. American Journal of Nephrology. 2005 Mar–Apr;**25**(2):154-160

[70] Hoyer-Kuhn H, Kohbrok S, Volland R, Franklin J, Hero B, Beck BB, Hoppe B. Vitamin B6 in primary hyperoxaluria I: First prospective trial after 40 years of practice. Clinical Journal of the American Society of Nephrology. 2014 Mar;**9**(3):468-477. DOI: 10.2215/CJN.06820613

[71] Fargue S, Rumsby G, Danpure CJ. Multiple mechanisms of action of pyridoxine in primary hyperoxaluria type 1. Biochimica et Biophysica Acta. 2013 Oct;**1832**(10):1776-1783. DOI: 10.1016/j.bbadis.2013.04.010

[72] Cochat P, Hulton SA, Acquaviva C, Danpure CJ, Daudon M, De Marchi M, et al. OxalEurope. Primary hyperoxaluria Type 1: Indications for screening and guidance for diagnosis and treatment. Nephrology Dialysis Transplantation. 2012 May;**27**(5):1729-1736. DOI: 10.1093/ndt/gfs078

[73] Stamp LK, Taylor WJ, Jones PB, Dockerty JL, Drake J, Frampton C, et al. Starting dose is a risk factor for allopurinol hypersensitivity syndrome: A proposed safe starting dose of allopurinol. Arthritis & Rheumatology. 2012 Aug;**64**(8):2529-2536. DOI: 10.1002/art.34488

[74] Torres RJ, Puig JG. Hypoxanthine-guanine phosophoribosyltransferase (HPRT) deficiency: Lesch-Nyhan syndrome. Orphanet Journal of Rare Diseases. 2007 Dec 8;**2**:48. Review

[75] Nicoletta JA, Lande MB. Medical evaluation and treatment of urolithiasis. Pediatric Clinics of North America. 2006 Jun;**53**(3):479-491

[76] Sahota AS, Tischfield JA, Kamatani N, Simmonds HA. Adenine phosphoribosyltransferase deficiency and 2, 8-dihydroxyadenine lithiasis. In: Scriver CR, Beaudet AL, Sly WS, Valle D, Vogelstein B, Childs B, editors. The Metabolic and Molecular Bases of Inherited Disease. 8th ed. New York, NY: McGraw-Hill; 2001. pp. 2571-2584

[77] Harambat J, Bollée G, Daudon M, Ceballos-Picot I, Bensman A; APRT Study Group.. Adenine phosphoribosyltransferase deficiency in children. Pediatric Nephrology. 2012 Apr;**27**(4):571-579. DOI: 10.1007/s00467-011-2037-0

[78] Gok F, Ichida K, Topaloglu R. Mutational analysis of the xanthine dehydrogenase gene in a Turkish family with autosomal recessive classical xanthinuria. Nephrology Dialysis Transplantation. 2003 Nov;**18**(11):2278-2283

[79] Brock WA, Golden J, Kaplan GW. Xanthine calculi in the Lesch-Nyhan syndrome. Journal of Urology. 1983 Jul;**130**(1):157-159

[80] Gargah T, Essid A, Labassi A, Hamzaoui M, Lakhoua MR. Xanthine urolithiasis. Saudi Journal of Kidney Diseases and Transplantation. 2010 Mar;**21**(2):328-331

[81] Mattoo A, Goldfarb DS. Cystinuria. Seminars in Nephrology. 2008 Mar;**28**(2):181-191. DOI: 10.1016/j.semnephrol.2008.01.011

[82] Goodyer P, Boutros M, Rozen R. The molecular basis of cystinuria: An update. Experimental Nephrology. 2000 May–Jun;**8**(3):123-127

[83] Saravakos P, Kokkinou V, Giannatos E. Cystinuria: Current diagnosis and management. Urology. 2014 Apr;**83**(4):693-699. DOI: 10.1016/j.urology.2013.10.013. Review

[84] Asplin DM, Asplin JR. The Interaction of thiol drugs and urine pH in the treatment of cystinuria. Journal of Urology. 2013 Jun;**189**(6):2147-2151. DOI: 10.1016/j.juro.2012.12.031

[85] Biyani CS, Cartledge JJ. Cystinuria-diagnosis and management. EAU-EBU Update Series. 2006;**4**:175-183

[86] DeBerardinis RJ, Coughlin 2nd CR, Kaplan P. Penicillamine therapy for pediatric cystinuria: Experience from a cohort of American children. Journal of Urology. 2008 Dec;**180**(6):2620-2623. DOI: 10.1016/j.juro.2008.08.057

[87] Nihon Asanuma H, Nakai H, Takeda M, Shishido S, Kawamura T, Nagakura K, Yamafuji M. Clinical study on cystinuria in children--the stone management and the prevention of calculi recurrence. [Article in Japanese] Hinyokika Gakkai Zasshi. 1998 Sep;**89**(9):758-765

[88] Pak CY, Fuller C, Sakhaee K, Zerwekh JE, Adams BV. Management of cystine nephrolithiasis with alpha-mercaptopropionylglycine. Journal of Urology. 1986 Nov;**136**(5):1003-1008

[89] Tasic V, Lozanovski VJ, Ristoska-Bojkovska N, Sahpazova E, Gucev Z. Nephrotic syndrome occurring during tiopronin treatment for cystinuria. European Journal of Pediatrics. 2011 Feb;**170**(2):247-249. DOI: 10.1007/s00431-010-1315-3

[90] Zheng Z, Xue Y, Jia J, Wei L, Shang W, Lin S. Tiopronin-induced membranous nephropathy: A case report. Renal Failure. 2014 Oct;**36**(9):1455-1460. DOI: 10.3109/0886022X.2014.926754

[91] Berio A, Piazzi A. Prophylaxia of cystine calculosis by alpha-mercaptopropionylglycine administered continuously or every other day. Boll Soc Ital Biol Sper. 2001 Apr–Jun;**77**(4-6):35-41

[92] Goldfarb DS, Coe FL, Asplin JR. Urinary cystine excretion and capacity in patients with cystinuria. Kidney International. 2006 Mar;**69**(6):1041-1047

[93] Chow GK, Streem SB. Medical treatment of cystinuria: Results of contemporary clinical practice. Journal of Urology. 1996 Nov;**156**(5):1576-1578

[94] Printza N, Koukourgianni F, Papathanasiou A, Augoustides-Savvopoulou P, Papachristou F. Efficacy of captopril therapy in cystinuria lithiasis. A case report. Hippokratia. 2007 Apr;**11**(2):83-85

[95] Conde Sánchez JM, Reina Ruiz C, Amaya Gutiérrez J, Camacho Martínez E, Vega Toro P, García Pérez M. Cystine calculi. Prevention with captopril. Clinical case. [Article in Spanish] Actas Urológicas Españolas. 2000 Feb;**24**(2):190-196

[96] Seyedzadeh A, Momtaz HE, Moradi MR, Moradi A. Pediatric cystine calculi in west of Iran: A study of 22 cases. Urology Journal. 2006 Summer;**3**(3):134-137

Chapter 3

Cystinuria: A Review of Inheritance Patterns, Diagnosis, Medical Treatment and Prevention of Stones

John A. Sayer and Fay Hill

Additional information is available at the end of the chapter

http://dx.doi.org/10.5772/intechopen.69984

Abstract

Cystinuria is a rare inherited renal stone disease. Mutations in two genes *SLC3A1* and *SLC7A9* underlie this condition, encoding proteins that facilitate dibasic amino acid exchange which are expressed in the gut and the proximal tubule of the kidney. Genetic studies now allow precise genotyping of patients who may have both autosomal dominant and autosomal recessive patterns of disease. The disorder is characterised by the urinary loss of cystine, lysine, ornithine, and arginine, and the insolubility of cystine gives rise to crystalluria and cysteine-containing renal stones. Although an inherited condition, it may present at any age. Clinical management combines lifestyle advice and preventative medical therapy. However, many patients require surgical interventions to remove problematic stones from the urinary tract. Preventative therapies include increased fluid intake, alkalinization of the urine, and the use of cystine-binding drugs, including penicillamine and tiopronin, which form soluble heterodimers with cystine.

Keywords: cystine, calculi, *SLC7A9*, *SLC3A1*, genetics, prevention, urine, crystal

1. Introduction

Cystinuria is an inherited metabolic disorder characterised by the abnormal transport of dibasic amino acids, cystine, lysine, ornithine and arginine, in the intestine and proximal renal tubule [1, 2]. In cystinuria patients these amino acids are excreted in excess concentrations in the urine due to a failure of reabsorption in the proximal tubule. Cystine is relatively insoluble; its presence in high concentrations in the urine predisposes to formation of urinary calculi, which are often large and can form staghorn calculi. On urine microscopy cystine crystals appear as flat hexagonal crystals [2]. The recurrent formation of the cystine stones can lead to development of chronic kidney disease [3]. Ornithine, lysine and arginine are more soluble and therefore their excretion in excess concentrations in the urine does not produce clinical sequelae. There are currently no known clinical consequences of impaired absorption of these four dibasic amino acids within the intestine.

2. Diagnosis of cystinuria: historical and modern

Cystinuria may present with renal calculi at any age, but most patients will present before 30 years of age. Historically, cystinuria was diagnosed mainly through renal calculi analysis and this lead to an underestimation of the incidence of the condition [1]. As methods developed to analyse the cystine concentration in urine samples it became possible to detect cases with confirmed accuracy, and also provided a valuable screening tool. The cyanide-nitroprusside reaction, developed by Brand et al. in 1930, provided a qualitative method of measuring excessive urinary excretion of cystine [1]. This test is positive when the urinary cystine level is greater than 75 mg/g creatinine [2].

Modern diagnostic methods may utilise a combination of laboratory tests, stone composition analysis, radiological investigation and genetic testing. Urinary cystine levels may be precisely measured using mass spectrometry, and are significantly elevated in cystinuria patients [4]. Levels of urinary cystine has also been used historically to detect carrier status, but a molecular genetic diagnosis is more reliable in the modern era. On urine microscopy, hexagonal crystals can be visualised which are pathognomonic [3]. Cystine stones are faintly radio-opaque and have a homogenous, ground-glass appearance [4], but may be missed on plain X-ray imaging. Cystine stones are often 100% cysteine but may contain variable amounts of calcium. CT-scanning allows accurate detection and localisation of cystine stones within the kidney and urinary tract.

3. Incidence and outcomes

Cystinuria is a rare inherited metabolic disorder, with an estimated incidence of 1:7000 live births [3]. The condition requires lifelong treatment, with the aim of minimising urinary calculi formation. However, the treatments involving high fluid intake, dietary modification, and urinary alkalinisation may be burdensome for some patients and compliance may be difficult. In those patients who continue to form recurrent cystine stones there may be an associated decline in kidney function over time [5].

4. Genetics of cystinuria

Cystinuria is an inherited renal stone disorder. Traditionally, a classification system based upon phenotype grouped patients as type I, II or III according to the levels of urinary cystine excreted by their parents, known to be obligate heterozygotes [5]. However, identification of the individual mutations underlying cystinuria, in addition to recognised limitations of the phenotype-based classification, has led to a new genotype-based classification system being introduced [6].

The heterodimeric amino acid transporter responsible for cystine absorption in the renal proximal tubule is formed by two proteins, $b^{0,AT}$ and rBAT, which are joined by a disulphide bridge [7]. The *SLC3A1* gene, located on chromosome 2, encodes rBAT and mutations in both alleles (homozygous or compound heterozygous) of this gene lead to type AA cystinuria. The *SLC7A9* gene, located on chromosome 19, encodes $b^{0,AT}$ and homozygous mutations in this gene produce type B cystinuria. Due to digenic inheritance of two or more mutant alleles there exist much rarer forms, including type AB, type ABB and type AAB cystinuria [8]. Such mutations account for only 2% of cases [7] (**Table 1**). Interestingly, patients with underlying mutations in *SLC3A1* and *SLC7A9* may sometimes present with calcium stones [9]. Genetic screening in paediatric stone formers may allow for precise diagnosis and earlier opportunities for therapeutic and preventative measures to be adopted [10].

Recently, a further membrane protein has been identified which is involved in cystine transport in the S3 (distal) part of the proximal tubule; mutations in the gene encoding this protein could account for further cystinuria cases. The AGT1 protein is encoded by the *SLC7A13* gene, and forms a heterodimer with rBAT to facilitate cystine reabsorption in the S3 part of the proximal tubule [11]. The discovery of AGT1 working alongside rBAT in the S3 section of the proximal tubule may help explain the previously recognised paradox of $b^{0,AT}$ and rBAT being predominantly expressed in different segments of the proximal tubule. It is known that $b^{0,AT}$ expression is highest in the S1 (proximal) segment of the proximal tubule, whilst rBAT expression is mostly in the S3 (distal) segment [11].

The clinical phenotype does not vary between the three recognised subtypes of cystinuria, although male gender and early age of stone onset have been suggested to be poor prognostic signs [1, 4]. As treatment options do not vary between genetic subtypes of cystinuria individual genotyping has not been routinely performed in clinical practice [4].

Gene	OMIM id	Inheritance pattern	Cystinuria type
SLC3A1	104614	Autosomal dominant and recessive	Type A and type AA
SLC7A9	604144	Autosomal dominant and recessive	Type B and BB
2p21 deletion	606407	Autosomal recessive	Hypotonia-cystinuria syndrome

Table 1. Known genetic causes of cystinuria.

5. Syndromes associated with cystinuria

There are three recessive contiguous gene syndromes associated with cystinuria. These are the hypotonia-cystinuria syndrome (HCS) [12], atypical hypotonia-cystinuria syndrome

[13] and 2p21 deletion syndrome [4]. Each of these syndromes includes the homozygous disruption of the *SLC3A1* gene, and therefore produce cystinuria type AA as part of their clinical phenotype.

Hypotonia-cystinuria syndrome arises from homozygous deletion of two genes, *SLC3A1* and *PREPL*, and has the least severe phenotype. The main phenotypical features are infantile hypotonia, poor sucking and associated feeding problems, growth hormone deficiency leading to growth restriction, mild facial dysmorphic features and cystinuria type AA [12]. Atypical hypotonia-cystinuria syndrome, which features disruption to three contiguous genes, *SLC3A1*, *PREPL* and *C2orf34*, produces an intermediate phenotype featuring mild to moderate intellectual disability in addition to the features of hypotonia-cystinuria syndrome [13]. The 2p21 deletion syndrome, resulting from homozygous loss of four contiguous genes, *SLC3A1*, *PREPL*, *C2orf34* and *PPM1B*, produces a more severe phenotype, as expected, owing to the higher number of genes affected [4]. Patients with 2p21 deletion syndrome may have neonatal seizures, severe developmental delay and lactic acidosis in addition to the typical features associated with hypotonia-cystinuria syndrome (**Table 1**).

6. Biochemistry and urine analysis

Confirmation of significantly elevated urinary cystine levels is key to establishing a diagnosis of cystinuria. The cyanide-nitroprusside test is a qualitative test traditionally used as a screening test for cystinuria; a positive result occurs when the urine turns red after the addition of the reagent, indicating a urinary cystine level >75 mg/g creatinine [2]. However, as the cyanide-nitroprusside test is designed to detect amino acids containing a free sulfhydryl or disulphide bond there is the possibility of obtaining a false positive result in cases of homocystinuria and acetonuria [4]. Precise quantitative measurement of urinary cystine levels is therefore always indicated in cystinuria patients, and homozygotes will often have grossly elevated levels of >300–400 mg/L, compared to the normal level of 30 mg/L [4]. In addition to measuring urinary cystine levels by mass spectrometry, urine microscopy may also be performed to look for the hexagonal colourless crystals which are pathognomonic for cystinuria [4].

7. Treatment of cystinuria

Cystinuria is an inherited metabolic disorder requiring lifelong treatment. In the absence of any specific treatment to reverse the abnormal dibasic amino acid transport, the target of therapy is to prevent cystine stone formation and thereby minimise complications of recurrent nephrolithiasis. Management of patients should ideally be undertaken in dedicated metabolic stone clinics [14]. Initial treatment is focussed on increased fluid intake, dietary modification and urinary alkalisation, but these interventions are cumbersome and patient compliance often limits their effectiveness. In refractory cases, a cystine-binding drug may be added to the treatment regime, although continued adherence to the initial conservative treatments is crucial for successful outcomes. Surgical intervention is reserved for large or symptomatic calculi which are causing obstruction, infection or pain.

7.1. Fluid

Maintaining a high fluid intake, aiming to produce at least three litres of urine per day, is the cornerstone of successful cystinuria treatment. Establishing a hyperdiuresis reduces the cystine concentration in the urine, thereby reducing the risk of nephrolithiasis [4]. The therapeutic target is to keep urinary cystine levels below 300 mg/L [15]. Nocturnal intake of fluid, both before bed and ideally at least once overnight, is an important factor, in order to avoid the increased risk of stone formation associated with the body's natural tendency to concentrate urine overnight [16]. However, it is hard for patients to comply with long-term [15]. Continued high fluid intake is a crucial factor in determining treatment success in cystinuria, both in isolation and in patients also taking thiol-binding drugs [15]; patient education regarding this is essential to achieve compliance with this burdensome intervention.

7.2. Diet

Dietary modification can help reduce the risk of stone formation in cystinuria. Patients are advised to follow a low sodium and relatively low animal protein diet. A low sodium diet is effective as dibasic amino acid reabsorption in the proximal tubule is partially sodium-dependent; a low sodium intake encourages reabsorption of cystine and sodium, thereby minimising excess urinary cystine excretion [4]. A low animal protein, or ideally vegan diet, is advised as this leads to a more alkaline urine being produced and also reduces the intake of the amino acid methionine, which is the precursor to cysteine [16]. Recipe books have been written especially for cystinuric patients that provide ideas regarding foods with high fluid content and low animal protein [17].

7.3. Urinary alkalinisation

Cystine solubility is increased in alkaline pH; a target urinary pH of 7.0–7.5 is recommended in cystinuria patients [16]. This can be achieved either by supplementation with potassium citrate or sodium bicarbonate, or through following a vegan diet. Potassium citrate is the preferred medication, but its use is limited in patients with chronic renal impairment due to the risk of hyperkalemia. It is important for the urine to remain within the target pH range, as over-alkalinisation can paradoxically increase the risk of calcium stone formation. Patients can use urine dipsticks to regularly check their urine pH [16].

7.4. Cystine-binding thiol drugs

Thiol-containing medications (penicillamine, tiopronin and captopril) can play a role in cystinuria treatment. These drugs bind to cystine in the urine, reducing the disulphide bond which forms cystine and producing two molecules of cysteine which are more soluble [4].

The use of penicillamine and tiopronin may be limited by their side-effect profile. Captopril, an angiotensin converting enzyme inhibitor, may be used as an alternative, although there is not strong evidence for its use in cystinuria [16]. Therapeutic success (reduction in stone events) is only likely to be achieved if conservative measures such as increased fluid intake are also followed simultaneously. Clinical trials using a new thiol binding drug called bucillamine are underway and will be completed by March 2018 [18].

7.5. Surgical therapies

Although stone prevention is the aim of cystinuria management, in cases where medical therapy has failed minimally-invasive surgical intervention can be required to break up and remove stones. This may be through lithotripsy (or extracorporeal shock wave lithotripsy), ureteroscopy or percutaneous nephrolithotomy [16]. These techniques are similar to those used for other types of renal stones. However, extracorporeal shock wave lithotripsy may be less successful in cystinuria patients due to the recognised increased resistance of cystine stones to fragmentation by shock wave lithotripsy [4]. Cystinuria is a recognised form of staghorn calculus which may require open surgical intervention and even nephrectomy in some cases.

8. Conclusion

Although a rare inherited condition, cystinuria remains an important cause of renal calculi. Establishing the diagnosis is crucial in order to prevent further calculi formation in these patients, whose treatment is distinctly different to patients with the commoner calcium-containing calculi. Our increasing understanding of the underlying genetic mutations causing cystinuria provides further information on the condition, and may eventually lead to treatments targeted at the underlying defect. However, at present, preventative medical treatment is the mainstay of treatment, reducing the calculi burden in cystinuria patients and aiming to avoid the risk of chronic renal impairment posed by recurrent calculi formation.

Author details

John A. Sayer[1]* and Fay Hill[2]

*Address all correspondence to: john.sayer@newcastle.ac.uk

1 Newcastle University, Institute of Genetic Medicine, Newcastle Upon Tyne, UK

2 Newcastle NHS Foundation Trust Hospitals, Newcastle Upon Tyne, UK

References

[1] Bostroem H, Hambraeus L. Cystinuria in Sweden VII. Clinical, histopathological and medico-social aspects of the disease. Acta Medica Scandinavica. 1964;**175**:Suppl 411:1

[2] Singer A, Das S. Cystinuria: A review of the pathophysiology and management. The Journal of Urology. 1989;**142**(3):669-673

[3] Camargo SM, Bockenhauer D, Kleta R. Aminoacidurias: Clinical and molecular aspects. Kidney International. 2008;**73**(8):918-925

[4] Pereira DJ, Schoolwerth AC, Pais VM. Cystinuria: Current concepts and future directions. Clinical Nephrology. 2015;**83**(3):138-146

[5] Sumorok N, Goldfarb DS. Update on cystinuria. Current Opinion in Nephrology and Hypertension. 2013;**22**(4):427-431

[6] Dello Strologo L, et al. Comparison between *SLC3A1* and *SLC7A9* cystinuria patients and carriers: A need for a new classification. Journal of the American Society of Nephrology. 2002;**13**(10):2547-2553

[7] Saravakos P, Kokkinou V, Giannatos E. Cystinuria: Current diagnosis and management. Urology. 2014;**83**(4):693-699

[8] Rhodes HL, et al. Clinical and genetic analysis of patients with cystinuria in the United Kingdom. Clinical Journal of the American Society of Nephrology. 2015;**10**(7):1235-1245

[9] Halbritter J, et al. Fourteen monogenic genes account for 15% of nephrolithiasis/nephrocalcinosis. Journal of the American Society of Nephrology. 2015;**26**(3):543-551

[10] Braun DA, et al. Prevalence of monogenic causes in pediatric patients with nephrolithiasis or nephrocalcinosis. Clinical Journal of the American Society of Nephrology. 2016;**11**(4):664-672

[11] Nagamori S, et al. Novel cystine transporter in renal proximal tubule identified as a missing partner of cystinuria-related plasma membrane protein rBAT/SLC3A1. Proceedings of the National Academy of Sciences of the United States of America. 2016;**113**(3):775-780

[12] Jaeken J, et al. Deletion of *PREPL*, a gene encoding a putative serine oligopeptidase, in patients with hypotonia-cystinuria syndrome. American Journal of Human Genetics. 2006;**78**(1):38-51

[13] Chabrol B, et al. Deletion of *C2orf34*, *PREPL* and *SLC3A1* causes atypical hypotonia-cystinuria syndrome. Journal of Medical Genetics. 2008;**45**(5):314-318

[14] Haritopoulos K, et al. Impact of a metabolic stone clinic on management of patients with cystinuria: 5 years follow-up. La Clinica Terapeutica. 2010;**161**(4):341-344

[15] Barbey F, et al. Medical treatment of cystinuria: Critical reappraisal of long-term results. The Journal of Urology. 2000;**163**(5):1419-1423

[16] Sayer JA, Tomson C. What I tell my patients about cystinuria. British Journal of Renal Medicine. 2016;**21**(1):17-20

[17] CystinuriaUK. Recipe Books. https://sites.google.com/site/cystinuriauk/recipes (cited 7 March 2017)

[18] US National Library of Medicine. ClinicalTrials.gov. https://clinicaltrials.gov/ct2/show/NCT02942420?term=cystinuria&rank=3 (cited 7 March 2017)

Section 2

Treatment Modalities

Chapter 4

Investigation of Laser Pulse-induced Calculus Damage Mechanism by a High-speed Camera

Jian J. Zhang, Rongwei J. Xuan and
Thomas Hasenberg

Additional information is available at the end of the chapter

http://dx.doi.org/10.5772/intechopen.69981

Abstract

Even though laser lithotripsy has become the most popular treatment choice for kidney stone disease, the mechanism calculus disintegration by laser pulse remains unclear. This is due to the multiple physical/chemical processes involved in laser pulse-caused calculus damage and their sub-microsecond timescales. A high-speed camera with a frame rate up to 1 million frames per second (fps) was employed in this study. The results revealed the cavitation bubble dynamics (oscillation and center of bubble movement) by Ho- and Tm-laser pulses at a different energy level and pulse width. Besides, fiber-tip degradation, damage, or burn-back is a common problem during the ureteroscopic laser lithotripsy procedure to treat urolithiasis. The results suggested that using a high-speed camera and the Schlieren method to visualize the shock wave provided valuable information about time-dependent acoustic energy propagation and its interaction with cavitation, the fiber tip, and calculus. And lastly, calculus migration is a common problem during ureteroscopic laser lithotripsy procedure to treat urolithiasis. In this investigation, calculus retropulsion was studied using a suspended pendulum in water to get rid of the friction. The results suggested that using the pendulum model to eliminate the friction improved sensitivity and repeatability of the experiment.

Keywords: calculus, cavitation, bubble, dynamics, shock wave, oscillation, high-speed camera, fiber burn-back, retropulsion, laser lithotripsy

1. Introduction

1.1. Cavitation bubble dynamics

Kidney stone diseases are crystallized solids, for example, kidney/ureter/bladder/urethra calculi or uroliths, which crop up in the urinary tract. The patient suffers acute ache and discomfort. Urolithiasis is the third largest disease in urology following urinary tract infection and prostate condition. It affects 10% of the US population at a significant recurrence of ~50% [1–3]. Shock wave lithotripsy (SWL) and the ureteroscopic laser lithotripsy (URS) are the top two most frequent treatment options in the USA for the treatment of ureteral stones [4, 5]. The review investigation in Ref. [6] concluded better stone-free rates (SFRs) for renal stones <15 mm for URS compared with SWL. Even though laser lithotripsy has become the most popular treatment choice for kidney stone disease, the mechanism of calculus disintegration by laser pulse remains unclear. This is due to the multiple physical/chemical processes involved in laser pulse-caused calculus damage and their sub-microsecond timescales (as listed in **Table 1**) and their timescales are very short (down to sub-microsecond level).

For laser lithotripsy, the laser pulse-induced impact by energy flow can be summarized in **Figure 1** as follows: [7]

- Photon energy in the laser pulse that includes the laser pulse train propagating through the delivery fiber and passing through the fiber tip (the fiber tip is typically uncoated and there will be a Fresnel reflection loss).
- Photon absorption that generates heat in the water liquid and vapor (resulting in super-heated water exceeding 100°C or a plasma effect with temperatures up to thousands of degree accompanied by light emission).
- Shock wave generation (at the initial injection of the laser pulse into the water. This is a Bow shock effect that results in an initial strong disturbance but dampens to a regular acoustic wave after traveling a fraction of a millimeter)

Effects	Thermal (heat up, vaporization, melt)	Light emission (plasma, super-heated water and stone particle, sonoluminescence)	Shock wave (supersonic, pressure shock)	Bubble dynamics (oscillation, center propagation, Acoustic wave)	Break (Chemical/ mechanical, fragmentation/dusting, spallation)	Kinetic move (debris ejection, retropulsion...)
Symbol				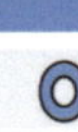	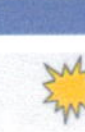	

Table 1. Physical and chemical processes during laser pulse-induced calculus damage [7].

http://dx.doi.org/10.5772/intechopen.69981

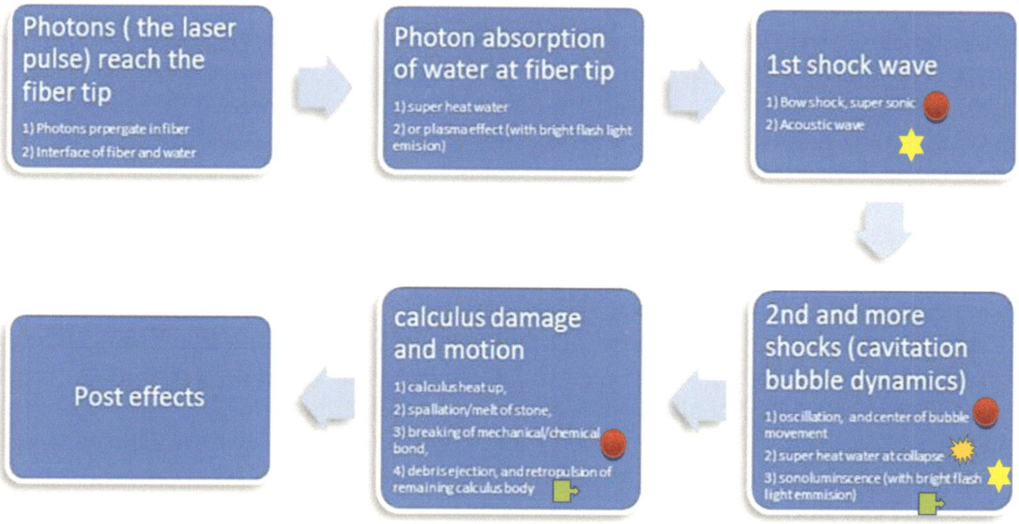

Figure 1. The energy flow block diagram of the laser pulse-induced calculus damage.

- Cavitation bubble dynamics (these include the cavitation bubble oscillation, the translational movement of the bubble represented by the center of bubble, the then super-heated water at the bubble collapse, the light emission by sonoluminescence, the shock wave created at the collapses of the cavitation bubble, etc.).
- Calculus damage and motion:
  i. Spallation: calculus damage through heating as the calculus rapidly absorbs the laser energy, thereby imposing a stress wave on the calculus surface. The magnitude of the stress wave and the temperature rise is proportional to absorption coefficient of the phantom; the high magnitude of the stress wave in calculus can cause spallation process;
  ii. Micro-explosion: the explosion of interstitial water content within the pores of the calculus;
  iii. Melt: direct absorption of laser photons by calculus that causes a temperature increase that exceeds the melting point of the calculus;
  iv. Breaking: breaking of the mechanical or chemical bond between the calculus molecules;
  v. Motion: includes debris ejection and retropulsion [8] of the remaining calculus body.
- Post effect (thermal dissipation across the calculus and through the surrounding fluids; debris spreading out by the acoustic waves, etc.).

Cavitation bubble [9–16] dynamics are the centerpiece of the physical processes that link the whole energy flow chain from laser pulse to calculus damage.

In this study, cavitation bubble dynamics have been investigated by utilizing a high-speed camera and a needle hydrophone. We keep the following three questions in mind when performing this investigation: (1) What are the differences in the characteristics of the bubble dynamics between a short pulse and a long pulse for Ho:YAG laser? A reduction of retropulsion and reduced fiber burn-back has been demonstrated by employing long-pulse modes in Ho:YAG lasers in contrast to short-pulse modes [17]. Several Ho:YAG laser vendors offer variable pulse option including the AMS StoneLight™ 30, pulse with a range from 150 to 800 μs. Indeed, it would be interesting to investigate the cavitation bubble dynamics as a function of pulse width; (2) there has been a dispute as to whether or not a cavitation bubble forms during lithotripsy when the fiber tip is in contact with the surface of the calculus. This contact mode is a common practice during treatment of urolithiasis and can be studied with a high-speed camera; (3) although Ho:YAG lithotripter is the benchmark for laser lithotripsy, the cavitation bubble dynamics and transient pressure level of other laser sources including the Q-switched (QS) Tm:YAG laser [18, 19] were also investigated. The study revealed the cavitation bubble dynamics (oscillation and center of bubble movement) and transient pressure levels of the Ho:YAG and Tm:YAG laser pulses at different energy levels and pulse widths. A more detailed investigation of the relationship between cavitation bubble dynamics and calculus damage (fragmentation/dusting) will be conducted in a future study.

1.2. Fiber-tip damage mechanism

The review investigation in Ref. [6] concluded better stone-free rates for renal stones <15 mm for URS compared with SWL. However, the delivery fiber employed in URS encountered distal-end burn-back [20–23].

As shown in **Figure 2** [11], fiber-tip (distal-end) degradation/damage/burn-back is a constant issue during the URS treatment of kidney stone disease. Fiber-tip damage leads to a decreased transmittance of laser power, which could lead to significant decrease of stone comminution. On certain occasion, the fiber-tip burn-back is so much that the degraded fiber tip will consume a lot of the laser power, which can lead to such a high temperature that exceeds the melting temperature of the fiber-cladding layer or polymer jacket. Although, it is a common

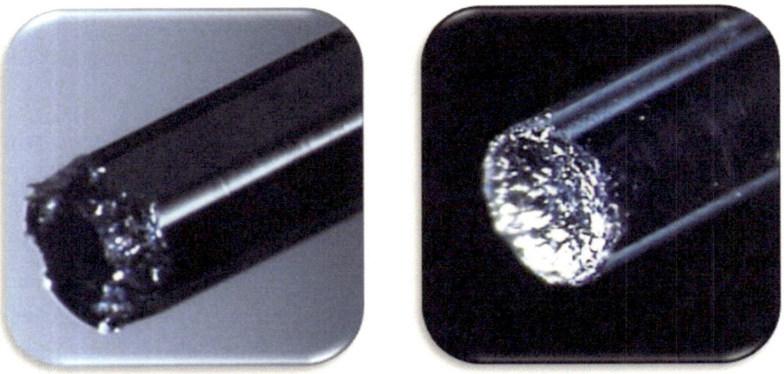

Figure 2. Samples of degraded fiber-end (burn-back).

sense that the bigger the laser energy density at the fiber tip, the faster the tip deterioration, the burn-back mechanism of the fiber tip remains unclear.

Fiber-tip damage/degradation/burn-back mechanism is a complex subject due to its numerous physical phenomena, for example, sonic shock waves, self-focusing of the laser beam, and transient thermal surge, and so on. It covers three areas of degradation mechanisms: (1) Mechanical: shock wave and debris impulsion; (2) Thermal: heating/liquidating of material, transient thermal surge because of the absorption of self-focusing laser beam by the microstructure of the fiber-tip surface material; (3) Optical: photoionization or plasma [24] as shown in **Figure 3**.

In this investigation, the fiber-tip damage was studied by visualization of the pressure wave, cavitation bubble dynamics, and ejected phantom stone debris using a high-speed camera and the Schlieren technique. A high-speed camera is a great device to study the relationship of the laser pulse with the phantom stone, as well as the recoil motion [8]. The principal chromophore of the 2.01-μm Holmium laser is water, which is critical for fragmentation of the calculus during laser lithotripsy [19]. The shock wave [9, 10, 12–14] that the laser pulse generates is a disturbance wave that travels faster than sound and is one of the mechanical causes of the fiber-tip damage (**Figure 2**). Because of the transparency of water liquid, pressure wave imaging inside water is not as straightforward. However, the Schlieren method can reveal the acoustic wave inside water, just like an X-ray which can reveal the invisible pressure variation inside a transparent matter. In this technique, a knife edge is placed at a focal spot to reduce the number of rays that do not interact with the acoustic field to reveal those that do interact; in physical optics terms, the Schlieren technique converts the phase information into an intensity image.

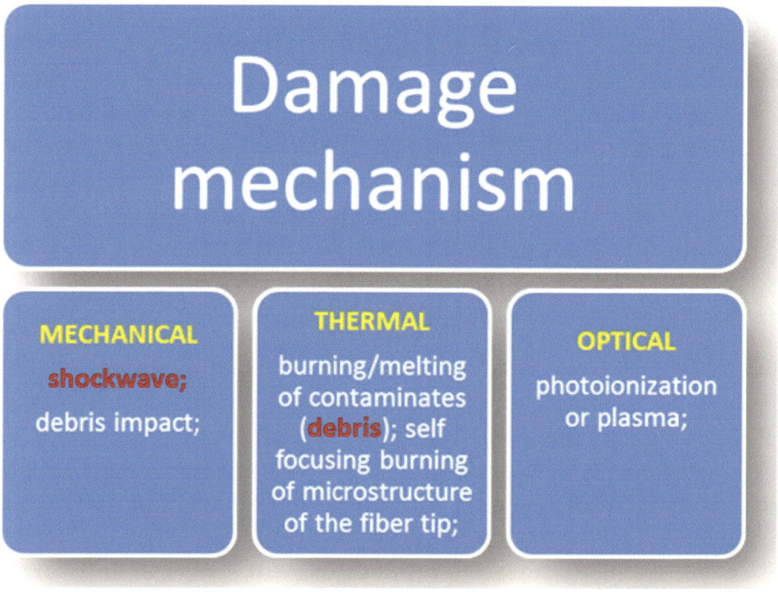

Figure 3. The degradation mechanism of the fiber tip (the items in red are studied in this investigation).

A commercially available pulsed Ho:YAG laser at 2.13 with a 365-μm core diameter fiber impinging on calculus phantoms (Plaster of Paris, white gypsum cement, 10-mm cube) was employed to simulate the URS process. Laser power-caused pressure wave, cavitation bubble dynamics, and calculus particles scattering were videotaped by a high-speed camera with 10,000–930,000 frames per second (fps). The pressure wave is captured by the Schlieren method. The contribution of ejected stone particles in fiber-tip degradation is also investigated. The study concluded that using a high-speed camera combining with the Schlieren technique is a powerful tool to study the movement of the pressure wave and its relationship with bubble dynamics and stone damage. More study in pressure wave shaping by the geometric shape of the fiber tip and the detailed mechanisms of shock waves, cavitation bubble dynamics, and calculus debris ejection will be investigated in a future study.

1.3. Calculus migration/retropulsion

During the treatment of urolithiasis, the urinary calculus is subjected to retropulsion forces induced by the combined effects of ablated particle ejection, interstitial water vaporization, and bubble dynamics [25–27]. Therefore, because of the retropulsion, the stone has moved away from the fiber tip. This can cause longer procedure time because of additional steps of finding the dislocated stone and repositioning the fiber tip to it. Recoil motion investigations in the past revealed the relation between retropulsion displacement and laser power, frequency, and fiber core size [28–31]. Recoil motion is proportional to the laser power and the fiber core size. Furthermore, another research claimed that the recoil motion decreased with a longer laser pulse without compromising dusting effectiveness significantly [32].

The amplitude of stone recoil motion (retropulsion) during kidney stone treatment depends mainly on the power source or instrument. The pneumatic or electrohydraulic lithotripters cause a much bigger recoil motion than laser lithotripters [30, 33–34]. Nevertheless, the laser lithotripters can cause noticeable dislocation of the stone during the procedure. A few investigations of the URS treatment of upper ureteral calculi have revealed that the main reason for calculus-free failures can be due to recoil motion and less frequently to inability to track or seek the stones [35–37]. Recoil-dislocated calculus could lead to longer operation period, the necessity for another process to deal with recoiled parts and as such reduced stone-free level. The stone recoil motion results in additional patient morbidity and health-care expenses [30, 33]. Besides, left-behind stone debris can act as a seed for calculus growing back, renal colic, and persistent infection.

The previous studies on stone retropulsion often employed a holder, like a test tube or a "V" shape groove. These approaches, however, have shown large uncertainty and low accuracy, most likely due to the friction between the stone phantom and the holder on which the stone phantom stationed. For instance, stone phantoms (Plaster of Paris, 10-mm cube) were employed to simulate the URS process, with the previous methodology resulted in <0.5-mm entire recoil movement (either with a "V" grove or a test tube). When scaling down the stone size to 5-mm cube (1/8 in volume), the recoil movement was very unpredictable. Our earlier study of recoil movement on a 5-mmcube resulted in a 59% standard deviation [38], for example, a peak-to-peak recoil movement range of ~3–10 times as much.

Sroka et al. [39] employed a sphere-shaped lead ball hung with a nylon string to investigate the recoil motion in URS by a standard CCD camera. In this investigation, a calculus phantom in water formed a pendulum, and the phantom recoil motion is studied using this approach to get rid of any friction that could occur if a holder was employed to host the calculus. This method mostly decreased the migration variation of recoil motion in URS. Furthermore, a high-speed camera was used to study the movement of the calculus which covered zero-order (displacement), first-order (speed), and second-order (acceleration) dynamics. This study employed a commercially available pulsed Ho:YAG laser at 2.1- and 365-μm core fiber, and calculus phantoms (Plaster of Paris, 10 × 10 × 10 mm^3 cube) to mimic laser lithotripsy procedure.

2. Experimental method and setup

2.1. Cavitation bubble dynamics

2.1.1. Fiber

Figure 4 shows a picture of SureFlex™ fibers, Model S-LLF273/365, 273/365-μm core diameter fibers (S-LLF273/365 SureFlex Fibre, Boston Scientific Corp., San Jose, CA, USA) that are used in the test of this study.

2.1.2. Calculus phantom

Calculus phantoms made of Plaster of Paris gypsum employed as tissue phantom for human calculi (UtralCal®30, United States Gypsum Company, Chicago, IL, USA), were broadly utilized for URS investigations by other investigators [40]. The calculus phantoms are made by mixing gypsum powder (500 g) with distilled water (0.23 l) and followed by curing for more than 3 h (preferred overnight). The gypsum was cast to have a dimension of 10-mm cube as indicated in **Figure 5**. The average weight of the stone phantom is 1.8 g, and with a tensile strength of 2 MPa, which is similar to the tensile strength of a human struvite (0.1–3.4 MPa) [41].

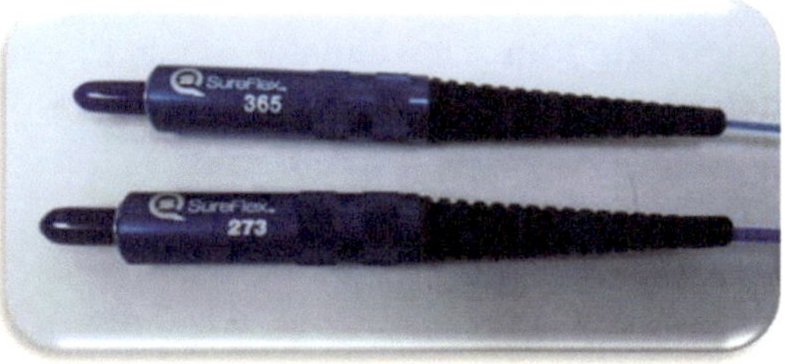

Figure 4. Picture of SureFlex™ 273- and 365-μm fibers.

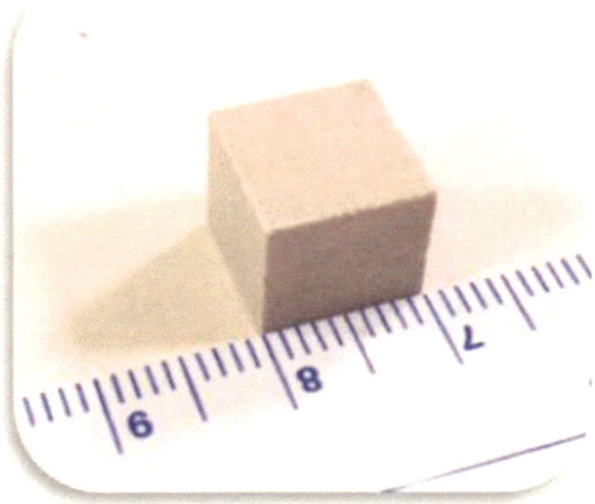

Figure 5. 10 × 10 × 10 mm³ calculus phantom.

2.1.3. Laser system

The laser systems utilized in this study included a pulsed Ho:YAG laser at 2.13 μm, Holmium 30 W (StoneLight™ 30, American Medical Systems, San Jose, CA, USA), with pulse energy from 0.5 up to 3.0 J, and pulse width from 150 up to 800 μs, as well as a Q-switched Tm:YAG laser at 2.01 μm with pulse energy of ~0.02 J. **Figure 6** shows a temporal pulse structure diagram of StoneLight™ 30 Ho:YAG laser with the pulse duration (τ_p) of ~240 μs. This magnitude of pulse duration is known to generate the necessary photothermal effect of fragmenting the stones [42].

A lab-constructed Q-switched Tm:YAG laser (2.01 μm) was used for this investigation, as indicated in **Figure 7**. The gain medium Tm:YAG is energized by laser diode pumping beam from a laser diode stack via a delivery system. An optical focusing glass is employed to compensate the strong thermal lens of Tm:YAG medium to sustain the stability of the resonator cavity. Besides, a lab-built acoustic Q-switch is oriented within the resonator to manipulate the output beam in a Q-switched manor. The laser has a frequency from 1 up to 2 kHz and pulse energy of 20 mJ at the distal end of the beam delivery fiber. Singular light pulse at the far end of the delivery fiber can be dispatched by an extra-cavity shutter in between the output window (OC) of laser resonator and the light-focusing optics system. **Figure 8** displays a light pulse with a pulse length (τ_p) of 750 ns (FWHM). This magnitude of pulse length is accredited to cause very intense shock wave pressure due to bubble collapse in water [13, 16]. This 2.01-μm wavelength light source is a suitable tool to study the dependence of water composition in the calculus on fragmentation effectiveness due to its level of water absorption constant at 70 cm^{-1} [43].

2.1.4. Setup

Figure 9 shows the schematic diagram and picture of the hydrophone setup: (a) schematic block diagram; (b) pictures of the setup. From the schematic block diagram, the centerpiece is the blue color water tank that hosts three holders with 3-D adjustable stages,

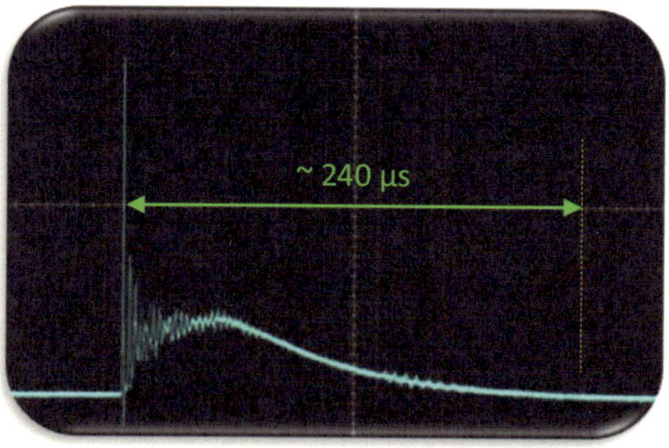

(a)

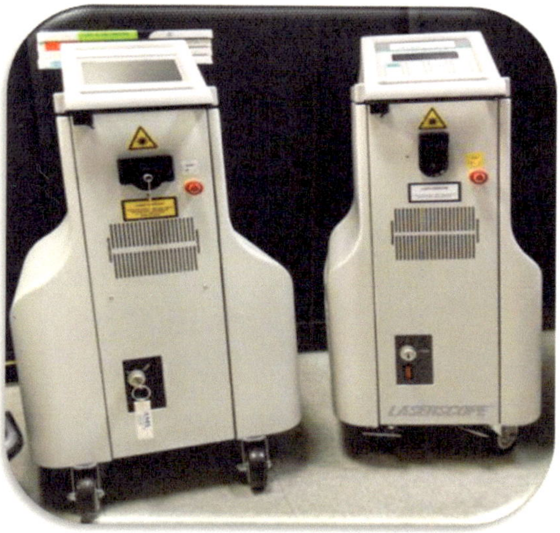

(b)

Figure 6. The StoneLight™ 30 Ho:YAG Laser system. (a) laser pulse trace; (b) Laser picture.

one for fiber (a 365-μm core diameter fiber, S-LLF365 SureFlex Fibre, Boston Scientific Corporation, San Jose, CA, USA, delivers the laser pulse), the second one for calculus phantom and the third one for the hydrophone (Mueller-Platte Needle Probe 100-100-1, Dr. Mueller Instruments, Germany). A ceramic screen is used to reflect the illumination from two high-intensity LED lamps for a better view of the action center near fiber tip. An SA5 camera from Photron (SA5 16G BW, Photron USA, Inc., San Diego, CA, USA), capable of one million frames per second, is used to record the event and the images are saved to the computer. The oscilloscope (Tektronix DPO 4140 Digital Phosphor Oscilloscope, Tektronix, Inc., Beaverton, OR, USA) is used to monitor and record the optical laser pulses detected by a photodetector (Thorlabs DET10D 2.6 μm InGaAs detector, Newton, NJ, USA) and the transient pressure signal from the hydrophone. In the hydrophone setup picture,

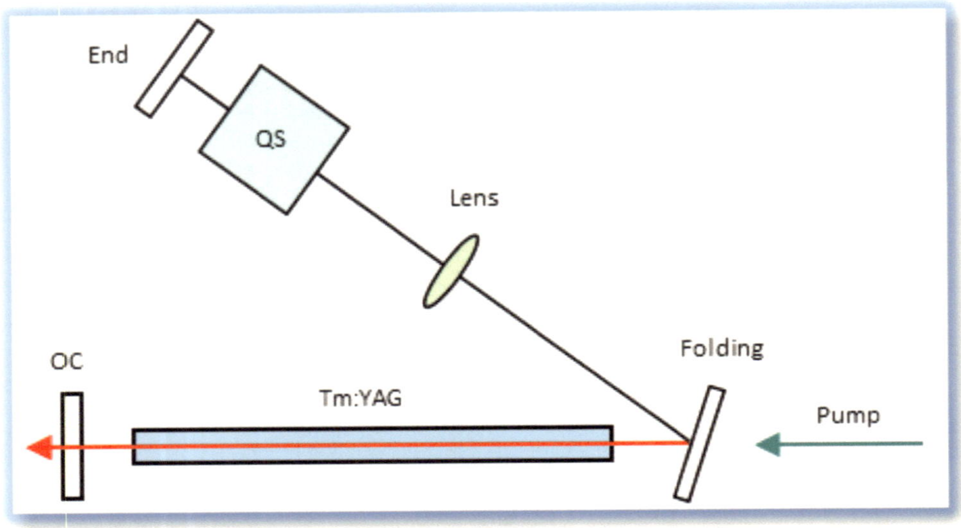

Figure 7. Lab built Q-switched Tm:YAG Laser setup.

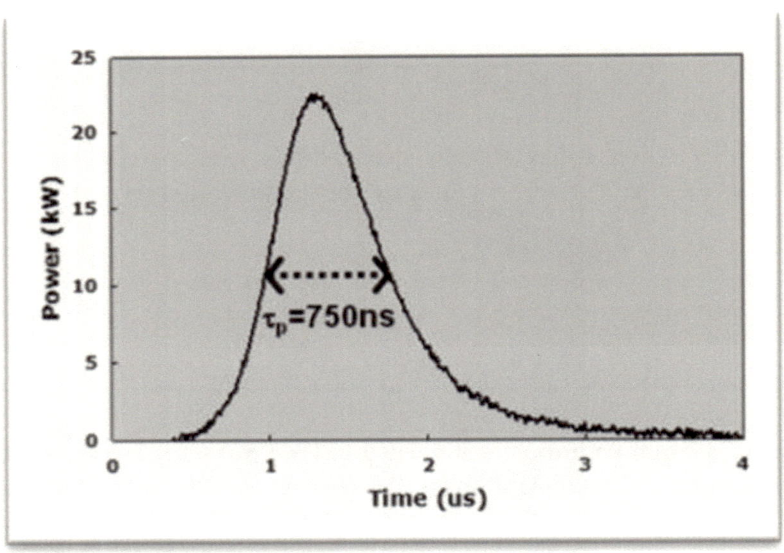

Figure 8. Q-switched Tm:YAG Laser Pulse.

it is shown that the tip of the hydrophone is ~10 mm away from the tip of the fiber. The hydrophone can be located at a different location or orientation if needed.

As a standard data collection convention, the entire test is repeated 10 times and each data point is an average of these 10 measurements.

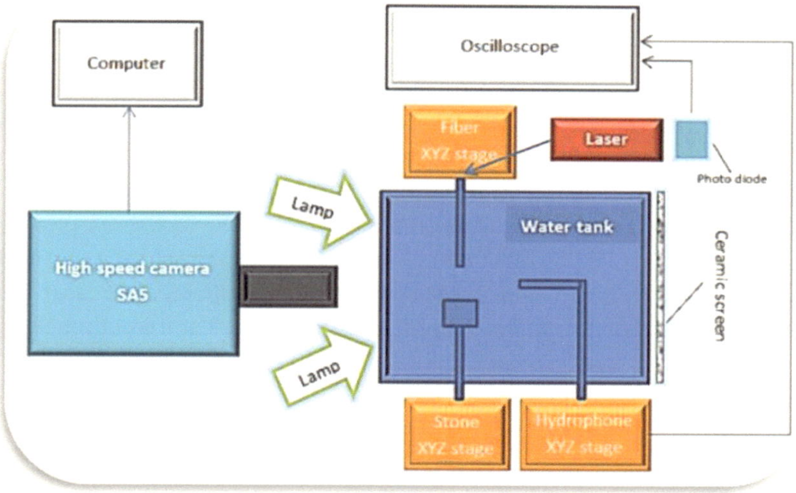

(a)

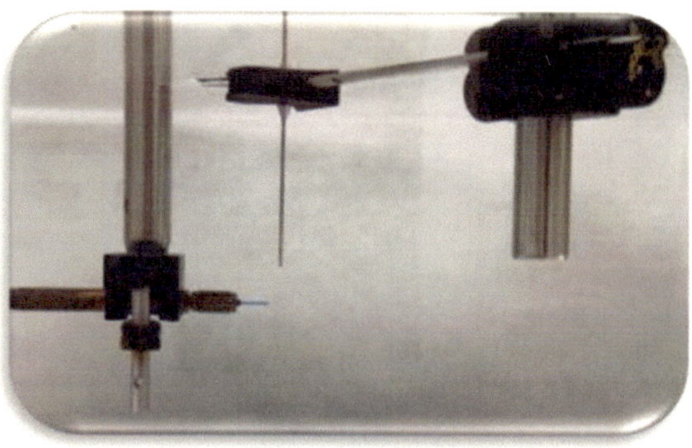

(b)

Figure 9. The schematic block diagram and pictures of the test setup. (a) Schematic block diagram; (b) Picture of the hydrophone setup.

2.2. Fiber-tip damage mechanism

2.2.1. Laser system

A commercially available Ho:YAG Lumenis VersaPulse® laser (VersaPulse® 100 W, Lumenis Ltd., Yokneam, Israel) was employed for this study. The laser is capable of generating 100 W of laser power at 50 Hz, and up to 3 J of pulse energy at 10 Hz. **Figure 3** shows a temporal pulse structure diagram of a typical 1-J pulse with a pulse duration (τ_p) of ~240 μs. Again, this magnitude of pulse duration is known to generate the photothermal effect necessary to fragment the stones [42].

This in vitro study again utilized a 365-μm core diameter fiber, and a calculus phantom (Plaster of Paris, 10 × 10 × 10 mm^3 cube) to mimic laser lithotripsy procedure. The test setup for laser-induced shock wave by the Schlieren imaging technique is depicted in **Figure 10**. The illuminating laser is a He-Ne beam at 543.5-nm wavelength. The two telescopes used for laser beam expansion each has a three times amplification. They enlarge the He-Ne beam size from ~1.7 to a 15 mm in diameter. The water box contains two handles with 3-D adjustable stages, one is for the fiber (a 365-μm core diameter fiber, S-LLF365 SureFlex Fibre, Boston Scientific Corp., San Jose, CA, USA) and the other is for the stone phantom. The focusing optics is a 100-mm plano-convex optics with a 2″ OD. The razor blade edge is positioned at the focus of the focusing optics. Besides, a high-speed camera was employed to videotape the laser-stone interaction. The SA5 camera from Photron has a frame rate of up to one million frames per second.

2.3. Calculus migration/retropulsion

2.3.1. Laser system

The laser system used for calculus migration/retropulsion is the same as that in Section 2.2.1.

2.3.2. Experimental setup

In this investigation, a commercial flash lamp pumped Ho:YAG laser at 2.13 μm, a 365-μm core diameter fiber, and a stone phantom (Plaster of Paris, 10 mm cube) were employed to simulate URS treatment process. An in-water pendulum is setup for recoil motion investigation, which

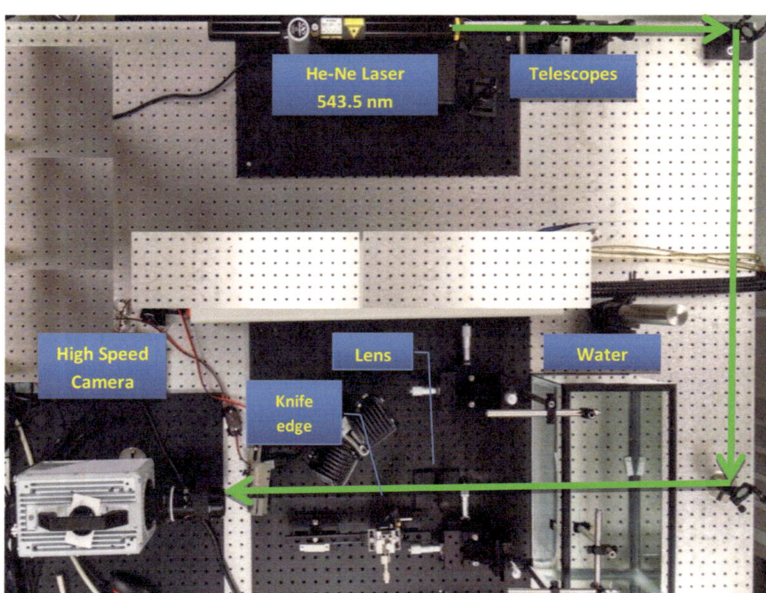

Figure 10. Schematic picture of test setup.

is composed of a calculus phantom with the size of 10 × 10 × 10 mm^3 as depicted in **Figure 11**. The calculus phantom is hung underwater by a string of ~200-mm long. In order to control the rotational motion of the stone in case the laser pulse from the fiber is not exactly pointed at the center of the mass of the stone phantom, the stone is held in a clear plastic basket and two threads with a separation of ~10 mm are used to hang the phantom (**Figure 11b**). Since water has a relatively low viscosity (1.002 mPa*s), the suspended phantom pendulum under water has virtually no friction and is free to move in the direction perpendicular to the thread. A 365-μm core diameter fiber (S-LLF365 SureFlex Fibre, Boston Scientific Corp., San Jose, CA, USA) was used to deliver the laser pulse to the stone phantom. Furthermore, a high-speed camera was used to study the movement of the calculus. The SA5 camera from Photron (SA5 16G BW, Photron USA Inc., San Diego, CA, USA) is capable of one million frames per second as shown in **Figure 11(c)**. In contrast to a conventional camera, the high-speed camera can be used to video tape and to fully characterize the kinetic motion of the stone phantom retropulsion. These dynamic details include the displacement, speed, and acceleration parameters of the stone phantom during laser lithotripsy.

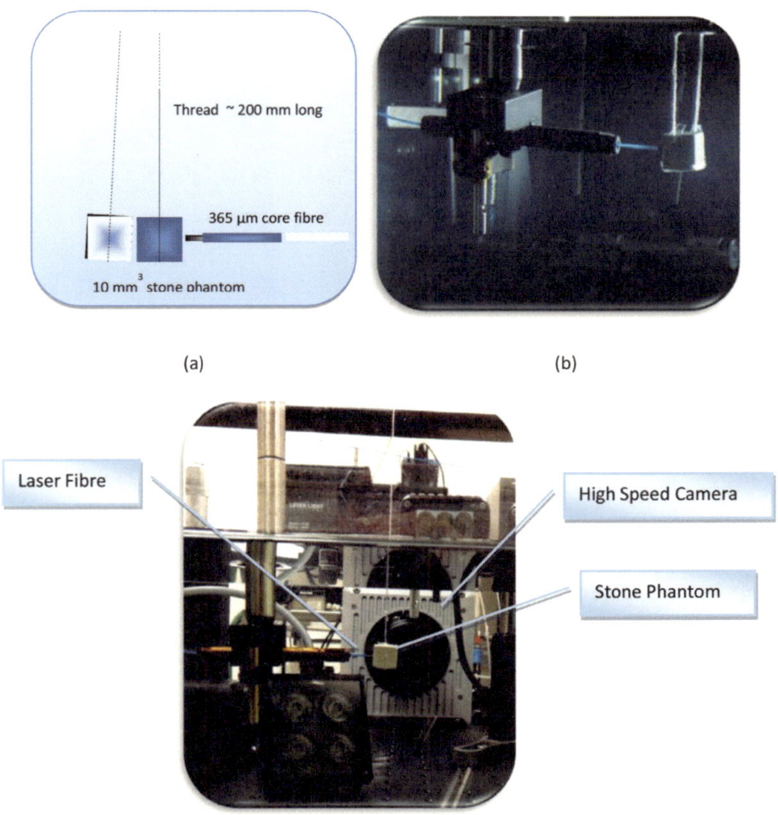

Figure 11. Schematic picture of the pendulum setup. (a) Schematic; (b) Picture of actual setup; (c) the experimental setup including the pendulum and high-speed camera.

3. Results

3.1. Cavitation bubble dynamics

3.1.1. Cavitation bubble dynamics in free running condition

The cavitation bubble dynamics was investigated by the aforementioned high-speed camera. **Figure 12** depicts a series of screen shots of cavitation bubble behavior created by the lasers. The Ho:YAG laser generated 1-J pulses with pulse widths of 150 and 800 μs. The Tm:YAG laser emitted 0.02-J pulse of a 450-ns duration. The high-speed camera SA5 was set at 300,000 fps with a viewing window of ~10.4 × 4.3 mm^2. As we can see from the pictures, the 150-μs pulse generates bubbles that oscillate up to ~3 times collapsing at 570, 773, and 902 μs. By contrast,

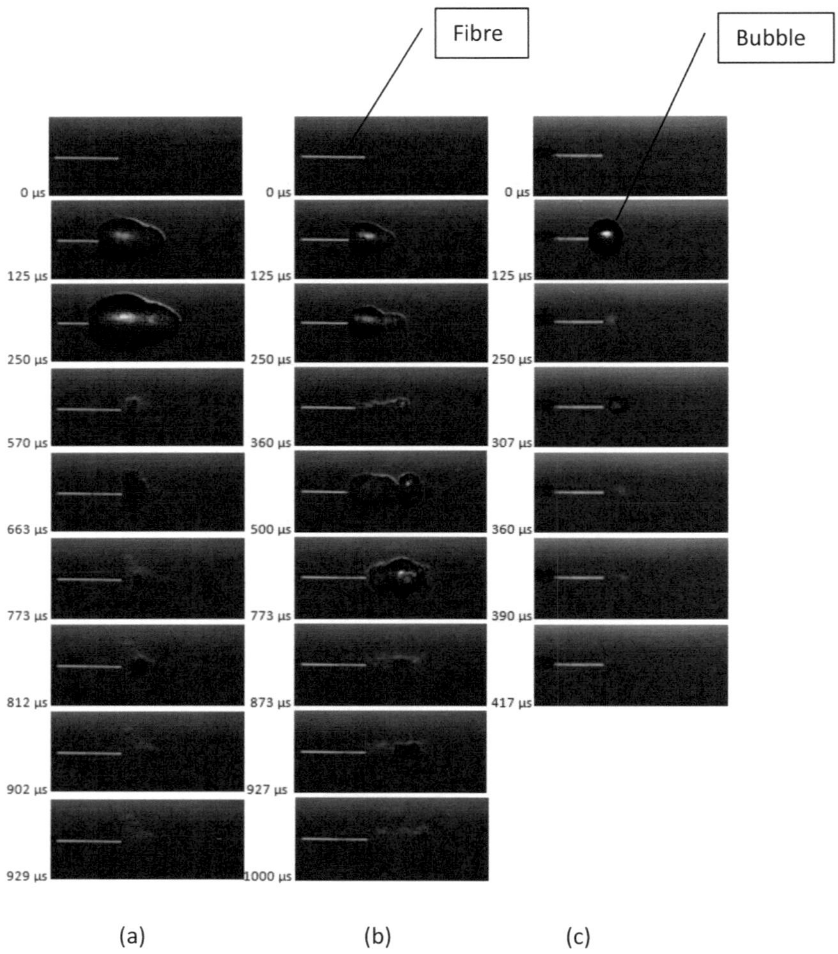

Figure 12. Series of screen shots of cavitation bubbles behavior of Ho and Tm lasers. (a) Ho at 1 J and 150 μs; (b) Ho at 1 J and 800 μs; (c) Tm 0.02 J and 450 ns.

the 800-μs pulse has a smaller overall size, and the bubble appears to have two parts that oscillate at different frequencies (see the first burst of the left part of the bubble at ~360 μs). Furthermore, the center of the bubble moves further away from the fiber tip (see pictures ~800 and 1000 μs). The bubbles generated by the Q-switched Tm:YAG laser have a spherical shape, and the size is comparable to those generated by 800-μs 1-J Ho pulses. Like the bubbles generated by the 150-μs Ho:YAG pulse, those generated by the Tm:YAG laser can oscillate to up to ~3 times as a single bubble. However, the time to the first collapse is much shorter (~240 μs).

Figure 13 shows the cavitation bubble oscillation curves. Each data point indicates an average of 10 measurements, and the error bar depicts the standard deviation. **Figures 13(a)** and **(b)** represent the 1-J energy level for the Ho:YAG laser pulses. The length is the horizontal dimension of the bubble and the width is the vertical dimension of the bubble. The bubble's first collapse is at ~500 μs, while for the 0.02-J Tm:YAG Q-switched laser pulse in **Figure 13(c)**, the bubble's first collapse is at ~240 μs. **Figure 14** shows the cavitation bubble center movement

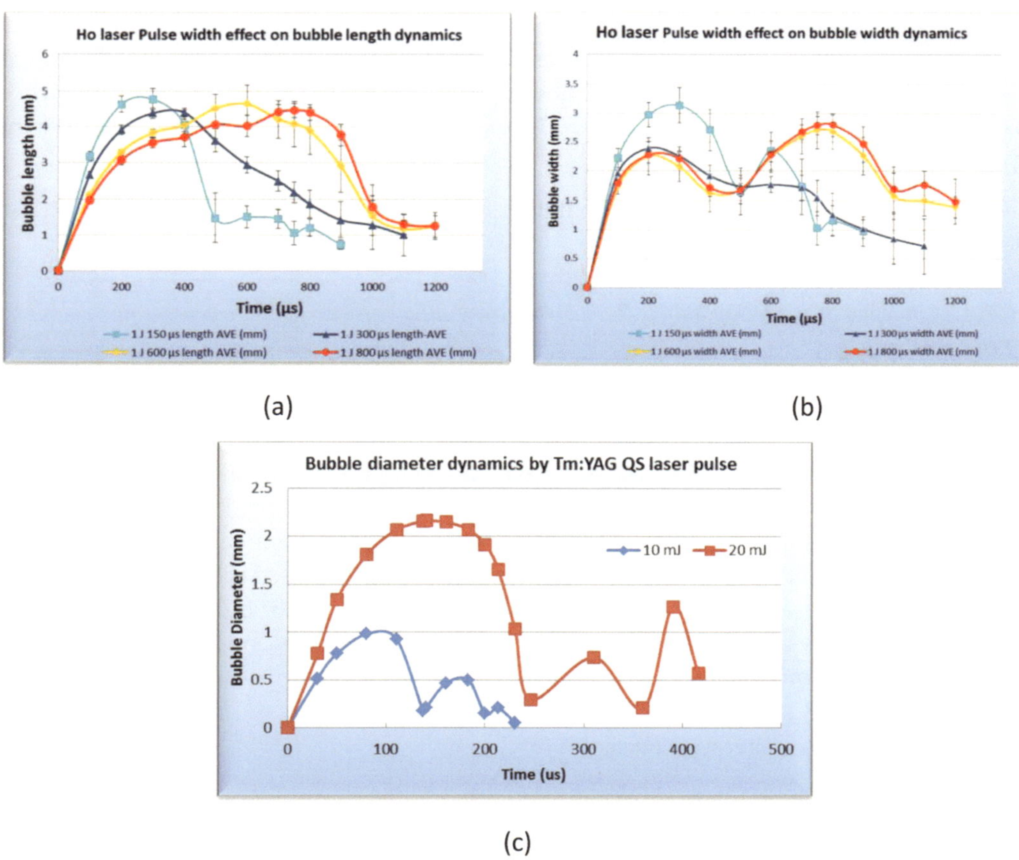

Figure 13. The cavitation bubble oscillation curves. (a) Bubble length oscillation curves of Ho:YAG 1 J laser pulse; (b) Bubble width oscillation curves of Ho:YAG 1 J laser pulse; (c) Bubble length/width oscillation curves of Tm:YAG 0.02 J laser pulse.

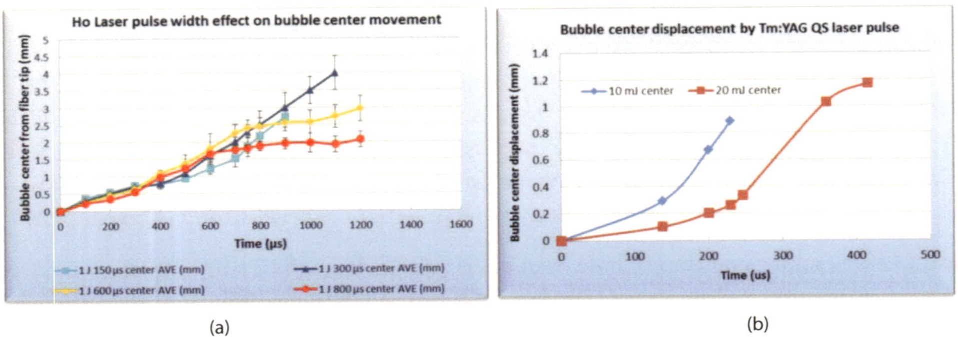

Figure 14. The cavitation bubble center movement at various laser pulse lengths. (a) Ho:YAG; (b) Tm:YAG.

at various laser pulse lengths. For the 1-J Ho:YAG laser pulse, at first bubble collapse of ~500 µs (this is typically the second and the highest transient pressure of the shock wave during the laser pulse interaction with the liquid fluid, while the first transient pressure of the shock wave is at the injection of the laser pulse as demonstrated in Section 3.1.3), Note that the bubble center is ~1 mm away from the tip of the fiber. By contrast, for the 0.02-J Tm:YAG Q-switched laser pulses, the first bubble collapse of ~240 µs, the bubble center is ~0.34 mm away from the tip of the fiber.

There is no observable difference of cavitation bubble dynamics between 273 and 365 µm fibers.

3.1.2. Dependency of cavitation bubble formation during lithotripsy on fiber-tip contact mode with the calculus surface

Next, we analyze the effect of contact mode whereby the fiber tip is in contact with the surface of the stone phantom. After analyzing the interaction video from the high-speed camera SA5 on the very first laser pulse hitting the stone, we observed bubble formation for both Ho:YAG and Tm:YAG laser pulses. However, in the Tm:YAG case, the bubbles can be seen more clearly because of much less debris generated by the 0.02-J pulse (as compared to the 50× stronger pulse in Ho:YAG laser case). The bubbles generated are hemispheres because of the existence of the stone phantom and the collapse time is shown in **Figure 15**. The bubble collapse time in contact mode is ~10–15% shorter as compared to the case without stone phantom contact for both Ho:YAG and Tm:YAG lasers.

3.1.3. Transient pressure level measurement

The transient pressure is measured by a hydrophone and its sensitivity $U_{probe} = Q_{probe}/C_{sum}$, where Q_{probe} is the 3.0 pC/MPa and C_{sum} is the sum of probe capacity including cable (244 + 13 = 257 pF); therefore, U_{probe} = 11.7 mV/MPa.

Figure 16 shows the oscilloscope traces of laser pulse and transient pressure. The upper picture has been created by a Ho laser pulse of 150 µs at 1 J and 10 Hz. The hydrophone end is

http://dx.doi.org/10.5772/intechopen.69981

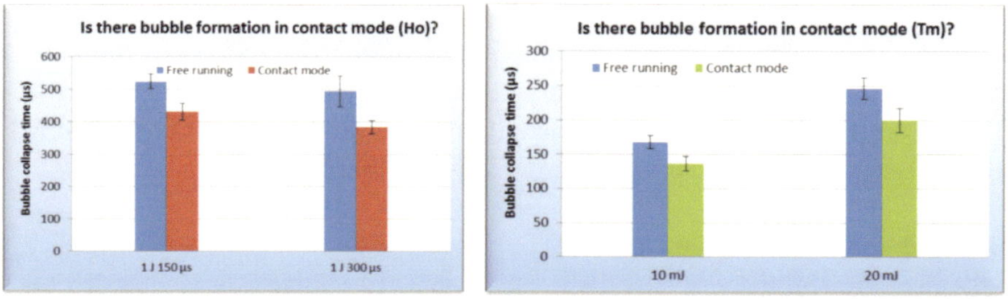

(a) (b)

Figure 15. The cavitation bubble collapse time in contact mode. (a) Ho:YAG; (b) Tm:YAG.

positioned at ~10 mm from the fiber end to prevent the probe from any possible damage due to the laser beam or pressure wave. Because the rising period of the hydrophone sensor is 45 ns, the detected transient pressure may be less than the real value. The actual pressure curve (**Figure 16**) exhibits many spikes, the first of which commences immediately after the injection of the laser pulse. This first pulse in the time sequence (from the left) represents the first shock wave. The second or the highest transient pressure peak corresponds to the first collapse of the cavitation bubble at ~500 μs. The average transient pressure is ~18 mV or 1.5 MPa at 10 mm away from the fiber tip. In addition, the transient pressure resulting from a 1-J and 800-μs pulse is less than half of that of a 150-μs pulse.

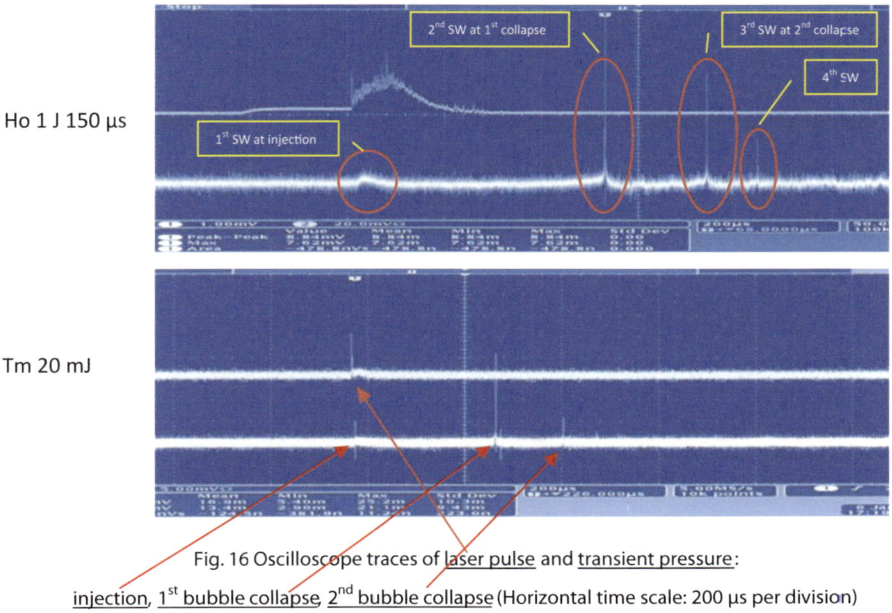

Figure 16. Oscilloscope traces of laser pulse and transient pressure: injection, first bubble collapse, second bubble collapse (horizontal timescale: 200-μs per division).

Similar sequences of transient pressure signals are shown in the lower picture, in which the first transient pressure by shock wave immediately after the injection of the laser pulse is more obvious, and the second transient pressure signal caused by bubble collapse at ~240 μs is again the strongest one. The highest transient pressure peak generated by a 20-mJ Tm:YAG Q-switched laser pulse is ~1.8 MPa at 10 mm from the fiber tip.

3.2. Fiber-tip damage mechanism

3.2.1. Shock wave detection

Shock waves generated by laser pulses are disturbance waves that travel faster than sound, but quickly damp down to the speed of sound [12]. The speed of sound under water is 1484 m/s or ~1.5 mm/μs; as such, a high-speed camera with a frequency of ~1 μs or 1 million fps is required for studying the dynamics of these pressure waves (with 930,000 fps, the period is ~1 μs, while the image size is barely a few mm wide).

Figure 17 shows a snapshot of the Schlieren image of shock wave by a 1-J pulse with a high-speed camera setting of 930,000 fps. In the picture, the captured image is at the moment when the shock wave (the area indicated in the middle) leaves the fiber-tip area and moves to the right.

Figure 18 depicts the shock-wave displacement curve against time. Utilizing a second-order polynomial curve fit, we can see the speed is 1.45 mm/μs or 1450 m/s. This is consistent with the sound speed in water (1484 m/s). However, the pressure wave is quicker than the acoustic velocity at the very beginning (within the 1-μs domain [12]). A well above 1-million fps frame rate camera is needed (best to be 10 million fps) so that a detailed understanding of the pressure wave initiated by Holmium laser energy can be obtained.

3.2.2. Fiber-tip damage

An additional set of tests were conducted on the thermal/mechanical damage to the fiber tip by debris by (1) varying the distance between the fiber tip and the calculus surface; (2) differing the incidence angle of the fiber to the calculus surface. According to a multicenter study of 541 procedures, the average dose of laser energy needed for laser lithotripsy is ~1.5 kJ [22]. Therefore,

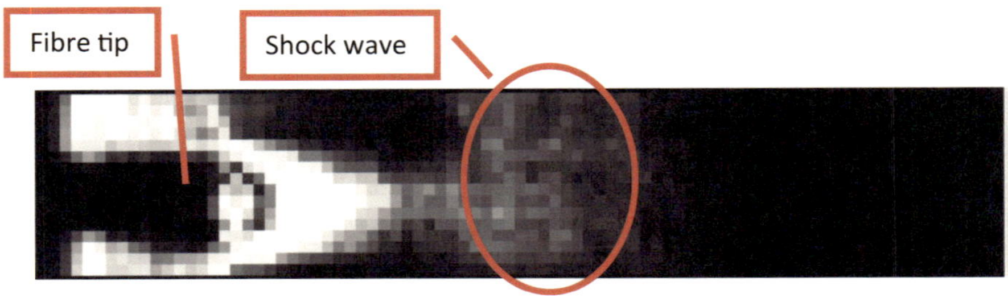

Figure 17. Shock-wave Schlieren image with a frame interval of 1.075 μs, and the frame size is 1.07 × 8.53 mm (16 × 128).

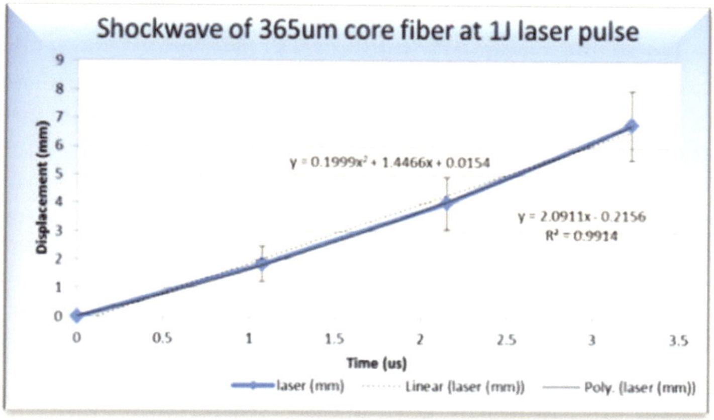

Figure 18. The shock-wave displacement curve against time.

a lasing time of 2.5 min (150 s) at 1 J and 10 Hz (which is equivalent of 1.5 kJ) is used for the damage tests shown subsequently.

Figure 19 shows images of the fiber and calculus with different incidence angles. In addition to varying the angular setting, the fiber tip is adjusted through a range of distances from the calculus (at 2, 1, 0.5, and 0 mm). Furthermore, the fiber is translated vertically at a velocity of ~0.4 mm/s within the 2.5-min laser on period in the same time holding a constant spacing from the phantom.

(a)

(b)

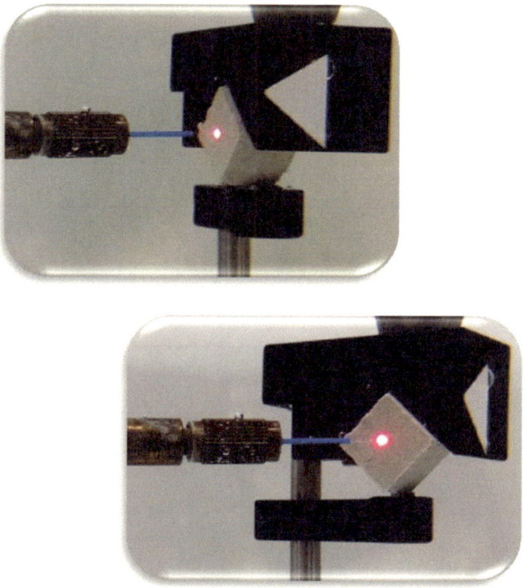

Figure 19. The images of fiber and stone phantom with various incidence angles. (a) 0° incidence; (b) 45° incidence.

In **Figure 20**, we show fiber-tip end views from fibers that underwent these various pulse conditions as well as an unused one. We utilized 1.5-kJ laser pulse trains at the four different fibers to calculus spacing (2, 1, 0.5, and 0 mm) and with two different incidence angles (0 and 45°). It is evident from the pictures that the fiber end surface damage/deformation becomes more severe as the separation between the fiber tip and calculus surface becomes smaller after 1.5 kJ of energy delivery. Besides, the 45° incidence angle results in less end surface damage/deformation verse 0° incidence angle for the same separation value. **Figure 21** depicts the transmission degradation of 365-μm fiber over working distance and an incidence angle after

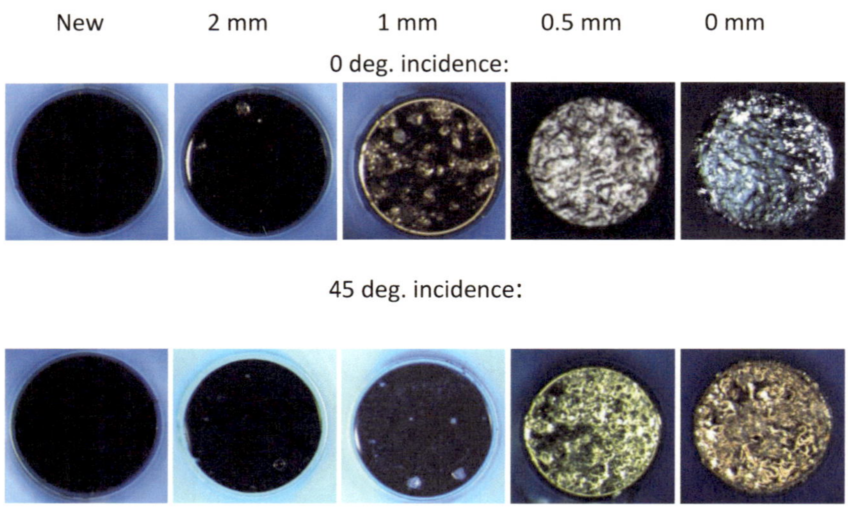

Figure 20. Fiber-tip end views from unused fibers in contrast to fibers after 1.5-kJ laser energy deliveries. Four different spacings (2, 1, 0.5, and 0 mm) between fiber tip and calculus surface, and with two different incidence angles (0 and 45°) were used for the activated fibers.

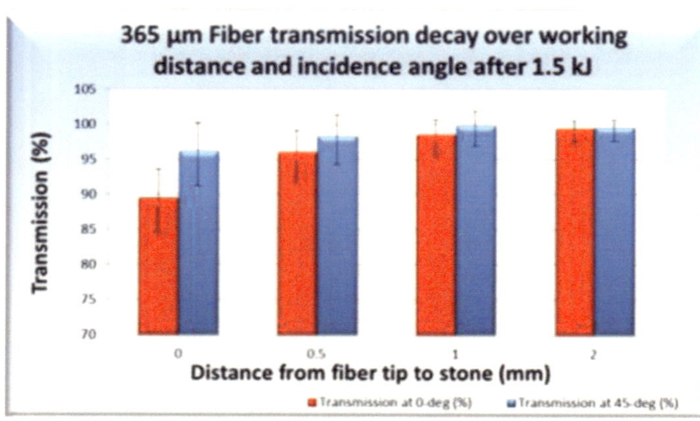

Figure 21. Transmission decay of a 365-μm fiber as a function of working distance and angle of incidence after 1.5 kJ of energy delivery.

1.5 kJ of energy delivery. The transmission measurement results are consistent with the surface damage/deformation results.

3.2.3. Retropulsion

Admittedly, our high-speed camera is capable of 1 × 10⁶ fps, but the field of view is limited at rates greater than 7 × 10³ fps. Therefore, we find that a frame rate of 1 × 10⁴ fps is a good compromise between speed and field of view for our retropulsion study. For each measurement, the high-speed camera recorded 10,000 images during the 1-s interval of laser pulses interacting with the stone phantoms. Each measurement was repeated 5–10 times to improve the data quality. The video data files are analyzed using a MATLAB program. **Figure 22** shows the pendulum retropulsion test at a 10-kfps camera frame rate and utilizing a Ho:YAG laser delivering 0.5-J pulses at a repetition rate of 10 Hz. Hence, 10,000 data points are recorded at these conditions and are shown as a dotted curve. This dotted curve depicts the zero order of the motion and hence the displacement of the stone phantom. The apex of the movement occurs after ~0.83 s where the phantom reaches zero velocity and begins to swing back. From this zeroth-order curve, we can generate the first-order curve (shown in solid) which indicates the speed of the phantom. We note that the initial speed depicted in the curve is not zero. This is due to the inadequate resolution of the measurement system. At a frame rate of 1 × 10⁴ fps, we have a 100-μs period between camera shots. This is too coarse compared to the 240-μs laser pulse since it will have a significant impact on the phantom within the 100-μs time frame. Lastly, the second-order motion represents the acceleration of the phantom and is represented by the Dotted-dash curve. The point that it crosses the zero acceleration line indicates the maximum speed of the phantom. Besides, the initial acceleration (multiplied by the phantom mass) is a good estimation of the average force that impacts on the pendulum by the laser pulse train within 1 s.

To further our study of retropulsion, we utilized our pendulum setup and employed various Holmium laser pulse energies impinging on a 200 mm–10 mm³ stone phantom. In **Figure 23**, we show the maximum displacements of the stone phantom as a function of laser pulse energy. The increase of apex or maximum displacement with laser pulse energy is to be expected. The

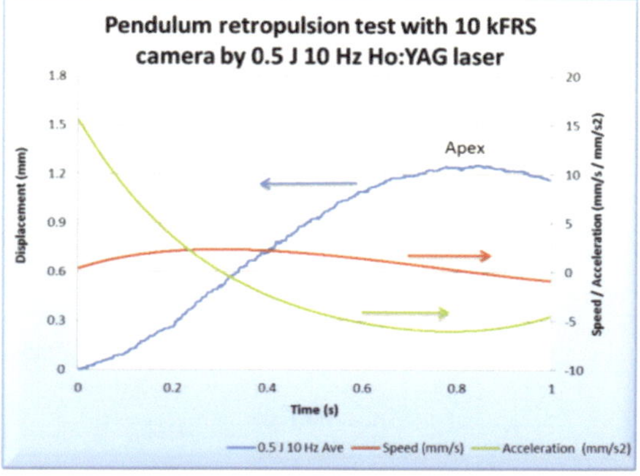

Figure 22. Pendulum retropulsion test with 10-kFRS camera by 0.5 J 10 Hz Ho:YAG laser.

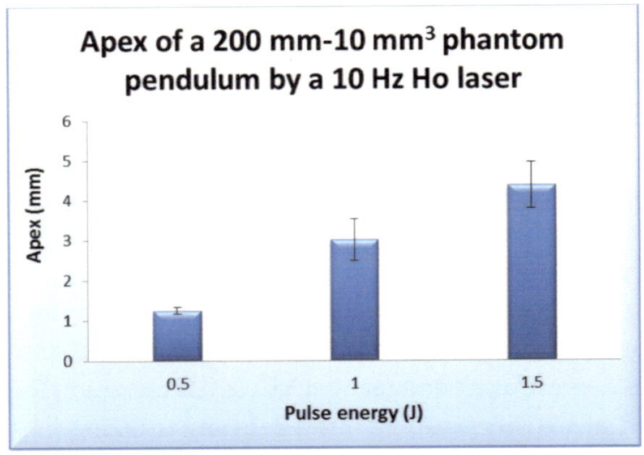

Figure 23. The apex of a 200 mm–10 mm^3 phantom pendulum by a 10-Hz Holmium laser.

results of displacement are 1.25 ± 0.10, 3.01 ± 0.52, and 4.37 ± 0.58 mm for 0.5, 1.0, and 1.5 J of energy per pulse, respectively.

From **Figure 22**, we can find out the initial acceleration of a 200 mm–10 mm^3 phantom pendulum by a 10-Hz Holmium laser at different pulse energy level. Taking into account the mass of the stone phantom ~2.0 g (wet and ~1.8 g when dry), the average initial force by 10 of the 0.5-J pulses is 3.1 × 10^{-5} Newton or 3.1 Dyne.

Figure 24 reveals the average power effect of retropulsion with the 0.5-J Holmium laser pulse train. Not surprisingly, the retropulsion increases with the average laser power applied. Apparently, the time to reach the apex increases with increasing average power. When the laser power level is increased above 25 W, the time for the phantom to come to the apex exceeds 1 s. This duration was beyond the high-speed camera recording time in our current study. In the future, further testing should be done with increased high-speed camera recording times (>1 s) to investigate the phantom dynamics at higher laser power levels.

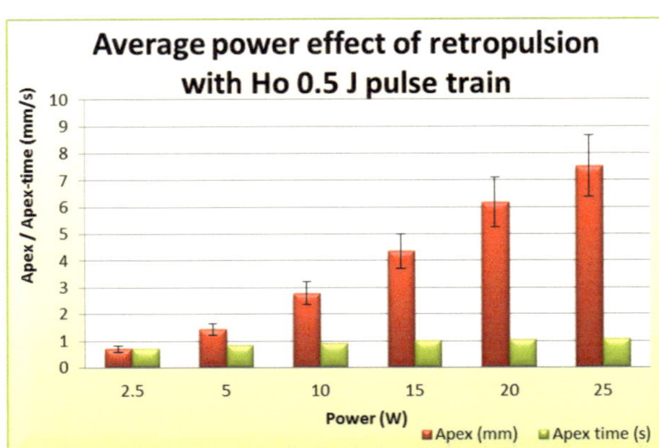

Figure 24. The average power effect of retropulsion with Holmium laser 0.5-J pulse train.

4. Discussions

4.1. Cavitation bubble dynamics

Urinary calculi are crystalline deposits, also known as kidney/ureter/bladder/urethra stones or uroliths, which occur in the urinary system. The presence of urinary tract stones often causes the personal severe discomfort and pain. Even though laser lithotripsy has become the most popular treatment choice for kidney stone disease, the mechanism calculus disintegration by laser pulse remains unclear. This is due to the multiple physical/chemical processes involved in laser pulse-caused calculus damage and their sub-microsecond timescales. Cavitation bubble [9–16] dynamics are the centerpiece of the physical processes that link the whole energy flow chain from laser pulse to calculus damage.

In this study, cavitation bubble dynamics was investigated by a high-speed camera and a needle hydrophone. We keep the following three questions in mind when performing the investigation:

1. What are the differences in the characteristics of the bubble dynamics when utilizing short pulses versus long pulses emitted from a Ho:YAG laser?
2. Is a cavitation bubble formed during lithotripsy when the fiber tip is in contact mode with the surface of the calculus?
3. What are the characteristics of the bubble dynamics for a Q-switched Tm:YAG laser [18, 19] in reference to the benchmark Ho:YAG laser lithotripter?

The results revealed the following:

1. The cavitation bubbles generated when utilizing long pulses have a smaller overall size (less transient pressure) and appear to have two parts that oscillate at different frequencies. The two bubbles are observed in **Figure 12(b)** wherein the first burst of the left part of the bubble is evident at ~360 μs and the center of the bubble moves further away from the fiber tip (action center shifting). We also observed that the transient pressure generated by a 1-J and 800-μs pulse is less than half of that of a 1-J and 150-μs pulse.
2. Bubbles are formed even when the fiber tip is in contact with the stone. The bubbles generated in contact mode are hemispheres because of the presence of the stone phantom. It was noted that the bubble collapse time in contact mode is ~10–15% shorter as compared to the noncontact cases for both Ho:YAG and Tm:YAG lasers.
3. The cavitation bubbles generated from the Ho:YAG laser pulses exhibited a football shape. By contrast, those generated by the Q-switched Tm:YAG (20-mJ) laser pulses were perfectly spherical. The size of the Tm:YAG produced bubbles is comparable to those of the 1 J at 800-μs Ho:YAG pulses. However, the time to the first collapse is much shorter (~240 μs) for the Tm:YAG bubbles and they can oscillate up to approximately three times as a single bubble. The highest transient pressure peak observed for the 20-mJ Tm:YAG Q-switched laser pulses was ~1.8 MPa at 10 mm from the fiber tip. This is similar to the peak pressure observed for 1 J at 150-μs Ho:YAG pulses.

The transient pressure trace by a hydrophone located ~10 mm away from the fiber tip reveals that the first shock wave appears immediately after the injection of the laser pulse. However, the second and the highest transient pressure peak corresponds to the first collapse of the cavitation bubble as shown in **Figure 16**. Since pressure peak can be much larger than the magnitude of the first shock wave, the latter is often overlooked. It should be noted that the first shock wave is more evident (higher peak pressure) at high laser pulse energies or short-pulse widths as present in the Tm:YAG laser case.

Finally, we observed no discernible difference of cavitation bubble dynamics when switching between 273- and 365-μm core fibers. This is most likely because the cavitation bubble dynamics relates more to the pulse energy and pulse width, as opposed to the pulse intensity. A more detailed investigation of the relationship between cavitation bubble dynamics and calculus damage (fragmentation/dusting) will be conducted as a future study.

4.2. Fiber-tip damage mechanism

Admittedly, a retrospective study in Ref. [6] revealed superior stone-free rates results for renal stones <1.5 cm for URS compared with SWL. However, the fibers used in URS as energy delivery devices often suffer distal-end damage. This is usually referred as fiber-end burn-back [20–23]. Fiber-tip burn-back results in a reduced transmission of laser energy, which significantly reduces the efficiency of stone comminution. Though it is known that the higher the energy fluence (which is the ratio of the laser energy over the cross-section area of the fiber core), the faster the fiber-tip degradation, the damage mechanism of the fiber tip is still unclear.

In this study, fiber-tip degradation was investigated by the visualization of shock wave, cavitation/bubble dynamics, and calculus debris ejection with a high-speed camera and the Schlieren method. The primary chromophore of 2.01-μm Holmium laser is water, which is critical for fragmentation of the calculus during laser lithotripsy [19]. The shock wave [9, 10, 12–14] that the laser pulse generated is a disturbance wave that is faster than a sound wave. Because of the transparency of water liquid, pressure wave imaging inside water is not as straightforward. However, the Schlieren method can reveal the acoustic wave inside water [15], just like an X-ray which can reveal the invisible pressure variation inside a transparent matter.

Laser energy-induced shock wave, cavitation/bubble dynamics, and stone debris ejection were recorded by a high-speed camera with a frame rate of 10,000–930,000 fps. The shock wave is successfully detected using the Schlieren imaging technique. The results suggested that using a high-speed camera and the Schlieren method to visualize the shock wave provided valuable information about time-dependent acoustic energy propagation and its interaction with cavitation and calculus. We successfully observed the shock wave generated immediately after the injection of the laser pulse. This "first" shock wave was also detected by a transient pressure sensor (hydrophone) as discussed in Section 3.1.3. By plotting the shock-wave displacement curve against time, we revealed that the acoustic wave speed that was more than 1 mm away from the fiber tip was 1.45 mm/μs or 1450 m/s. This is comparable to the sound speed in water (1484 m/s). Furthermore, it is in good agreement with Ref. [12] that indicates shock waves only exist within a millimeter of the fiber tip and

http://dx.doi.org/10.5772/intechopen.69981

travel faster than the sound speed. Therefore, in the current study that utilized a high-speed camera with a frame rate of 1 million fps, or 1 μs per frame, the acoustic wave will travel 1.48 mm during a camera frame. Apparently, a high-speed camera with frame rate well at or near 10 million fps is desired to resolve more detail of the shock-wave dynamics generated by laser pulses.

The role of debris in fiber-tip damage is also studied. Fiber-tip damage/degradation/burn-back mechanism is an intricate subject due to its numerous physical phenomena, for example, sonic shock waves, self-focusing of the laser beam, and transient thermal surge, and so on. It covers three areas of degradation mechanisms:

1. Mechanical: shock wave and debris impulsion;
2. Thermal: heating/liquidating of material, transient thermal surge because of the absorption of self-focusing laser beam by the microstructure of the fiber-tip surface material;
3. Optical: photoionization or plasma [24].

The function of the stone particle in fiber-tip degradation mechanism has two folds: kinetic impulsion and thermal heating/melting. **Figure 25** depicts the stone particle clusters hovering around the fiber-end area and the fiber-end degradation/deformation after 1.5-kJ laser power dose and laser-stone interaction in our test. Our investigation reveals that the fiber-tip degradation/deformation is more significant when the spacing between the fiber end and stone surface is less. And with similar spacing, the 45° incidence angle leads to less tip surface degradation/deformation as compared to 0° incidence ones.

More investigation should be performed to find out the predominant degradation mechanism by the stone particle (thermal or kinetic), cavitation bubble dynamics, and balance between degradation/burn-back control and the stone dusting efficiency.

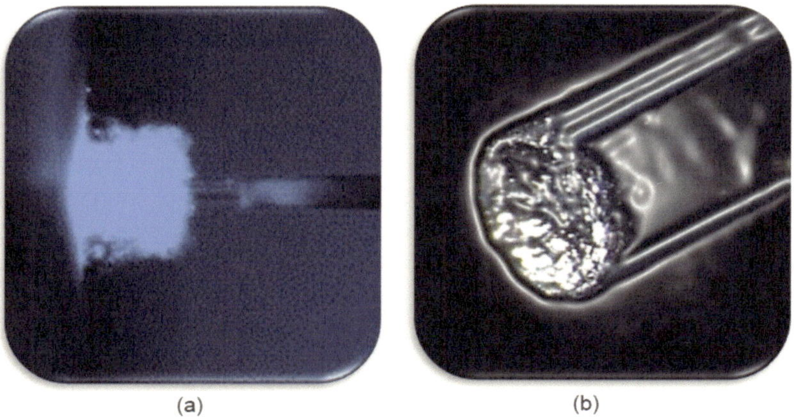

Figure 25. The stone particle clusters hovering around the fiber-end area (a) and the fiber-end degradation/deformation after 1.5-kJ laser power dose and laser-stone interaction (b).

4.3. Calculus migration/retropulsion

A few investigations of the URS treatment of upper ureteral calculi have revealed that the main reason for calculus-free failures can be due to recoil motion and less frequently to inability to track or seek the stones [35–37]. Recoil-dislocated calculus could lead to longer operation period, the necessity for another process to deal with recoiled parts and as such reduced stone-free level. The stone recoil motion results in additional patient morbidity and healthcare expenses [30, 33]. Besides, left-behind stone debris can act as a seed for calculus growing back, renal colic, and persistent infection.

Recoil motion investigations in the past revealed the relation between retropulsion displacement and laser power, frequency, and fiber core size [28–31]. Recoil motion is proportional to the laser power and the fiber core size. Furthermore, another research claimed that the recoil motion decreased with a longer laser pulse without compromising dusting effectiveness significantly [32]. A conventional experimental method to characterize calculus migration utilized a hosting container (e.g., a "V" groove, a flat and smooth surface, or a test tube). These methods, however, demonstrated large variation and poor detectability, possibly attributing to friction between the calculus and the container on which the calculus was situated. Our earlier study of retropulsion [38] and Blackmon et al. [44] showed more than 100% the peak-to-peak retropulsion variation with the conventional experimental method.

Sroka et al. [39] used a ball-shaped lead sinker fixed to a nylon string to study the retropulsion during laser lithotripsy with a regular CCD camera. In this in vitro study, a high-speed camera was used to study the movement of the calculus which covered displacement, speed, and acceleration. Our study shows that the combination of a pendulum and a high-speed camera provides a very useful tool for retropulsion characterization. The apexes of a 200 mm–10 mm^3 phantom pendulum by a 10-Hz Holmium laser are 1.25 ± 0.10, 3.01 ± 0.52, and 4.37 ± 0.58 mm for 0.5-, 1.0-, and 1.5-J energy per pulse, respectively (peak-to-peak variation is less than 50%). And the average initial force by 10 of 0.5-J pulses is 3.1×10^{-5} Newton or 3.1 Dyne. These data conclude that utilizing a pendulum method to get rid of the friction enhanced the detectability and repeatability, and the high-speed camera provides a better understanding of laser-calculus interaction, especially the recoil motion of the calculus and its particles, cavitation bubble forming and burst, and so on.

Even though URS is now the top treatment choice for urolithiasis, further investigation should be done to gain a thorough knowledge of the detailed processes during the laser-water and laser-stone interactions. At least four processes play a role in the URS: (1) heat (super-heated water or sometimes plasma formation); (2) acoustic or pressure wave (cavitation bubble forming and burst); (3) chemical (disintegrate of mechanical and chemical bond between the calculus particles); (4) physical kinetic (recoil motion of the calculus and scattering of the particles). The high-speed camera combined with a calculus pendulum can provide a better understanding of items 2 and 4. More investigation should be conducted on all of the four processes of the laser-calculus interactions in the URS.

In summary, combining a high-speed camera with other tools/method: hydrophone, pendulum, and Schlieren imaging method, provides not only a very useful tool for cavitation bubble, shock wave, fiber burn-back, and retropulsion characterization but also a great insight into laser-calculus interaction in regard to acoustic and kinetic processes.

Acknowledgements

The authors thank Jason Gong, Xirong Yang, and Joanne Banuelos of Boston Scientific Corporation for their assistance with preparing the Tm:YAG Q-switched laser and tissue phantoms. Besides, we thank David Jebens of Boston Scientific Corporation for his help in capturing the fiber-tip images using Leica M205C Stereo Microscope. Final thanks extend to Grant Getzan of Boston Scientific Corporation for his assistance with the experiments.

Author details

Jian J. Zhang*, Rongwei J. Xuan and Thomas Hasenberg

*Address all correspondence to: james.zhang@bsci.com

Boston Scientific Corporation, San Jose, California, USA

References

[1] Matlaga BR, Jansen JP, Meckley LM, Byrne TW, Lingeman JE. Economic outcomes of treatment for ureteral and renal stones: A systematic literature review. Journal of Urology. 2012;**188**(8):449-454

[2] Rizvi SAH, Naqvi SAA, Hussain Z, Hashmi A, Hussain M, Zafar MN, Mehdi H, Khalid R. The management of stone disease. BJU International. 2002;**89**(Supplement 1):62-68

[3] Tiselius H-G. Epidemiology and medical management of stone disease. BJU International. 2003;**91**:758-767

[4] Pearle MS, Calhoun EA, Curhan GC. Urologic Diseases of America Project. Urologic diseases in America project: Urolithiasis. Journal of Urology. 2005;**173**:848-857

[5] Stephan Seklehner Meliswa A, Del Pizzo LJ, Chughtai B, Lee RK. Renal calculi: Trends in the utilization of shockwave lithotripsy and ureteroscopy. The Canadian Journal of Urology. 2015;**22**(1):7627-7634

[6] Cone EB, Eisner BH, Ursiny M, Pareek G. Cost-effectiveness comparison of renal calculi treated with ureteroscopic laser lithotripsy versus shockwave lithotripsy. Journal of Endourology. 2014;**28**(6):639-643

[7] Zhang JJ, Xuan JR, Yu H, Devincentis D. Study of cavitation bubble dynamics during Ho:YAG laser lithotripsy by high-speed camera. In: Proceedings of SPIE. Vol. **9689**. Photonic Therapeutics and Diagnostics XII. 96891E. San Francisco, California, USA: SPIE; 2016. P. 1-7

[8] Zhang JJ, Rajabhandharaks D, Xuan JR, Chia RWJ, Hasenberg T. Characterization of calculus migration during Ho:YAG laser lithotripsy by high speed camera using

suspended pendulum method. In: Proceedings of SPIE. Vol. **8926**. Photonic Therapeutics and Diagnostics X. 89261I. San Francisco, California, USA: SPIE; 2014. P. 1-7

[9] Akhatov I, Lindau O, Topolnikov A, Mettin R, Vakhitova N, Lauterborn W. Collapse and rebound of a laser-induced cavitation bubble. Physics of Fluids. 2002;**13**(10):2805-2819

[10] Johnsena E, Colonius T. Shock-induced collapse of a gas bubble in shockwave lithotripsy. Journal of Acoustic Society of America. 2008;**124**(4):2011-2020

[11] Zhang JJ, Getzan G, Xuan JR, Yu H. Study of fibre-tip damage mechanism during Ho:YAG laser lithotripsy by high-speed camera and the Schlieren method. In: Proceedings of SPIE. Vol. **9303.** Photonic Therapeutics and Diagnostics XI. 930311. San Francisco, California, USA: SPIE; 2015. P. 1-10

[12] Lauterborn W, Vogel A. shockwave emission by laser generated bubbles. In: Delale CF, editor. Bubble Dynamics & Shock Waves. Springer-Verlag; Shockwaves. 2013;**8**:67-103

[13] Zhong P, Tong H-L, Cocks FH, Pearle MS, Preminger GM. Transient cavitation and acoustic emission produced by different laser lithotripters. Journal of Endourology. 1998;**12**(4):371-378

[14] Lee H, Gojani AB, Han T-H, Yoh JJ. Dynamics of laser-induced bubble collapse visualized by time-resolved optical shadowgraph. Journal of Vision. 2011;**14**:331-337

[15] Korpel A, Mehrl D, Lin HH. Schlieren imaging of sound fields. In: IEEE 1987 Ultrasonics Symposium. Denver, Colorado, USA: IEEE; 1987. p.515-518

[16] Jansen ED, Asshauer T, Frenz M, Motamedi M, Delacretaz G, Welch AJ. Effect of pulse duration on bubble formation and laser-induced pressure waves during Holmium laser ablation. Lasers in Surgery and Medicine. 1996;**18**(3):278-293

[17] Sroka R, Pongratz T, Scheib G, Khoder W, Stief CG, Herrmann T, Nagele U, Bader MJ. Impact of pulse duration on Ho:YAG laser lithotripsy: Treatment aspects on the single-pulse level. World Journal of Urology. 2015;**33**:479-485

[18] Zhang JJ, Rajabhandharaks D, Xuan JR, Wang H, Chia RWJ, Hasenberg T, Kang HW. Water content contribution in calculus phantomablation during Q-switched Tm:YAG laser lithotripsy. Journal of Biomedical Optics. 2015;**20**(12):128001

[19] Rajabhandharaks D, Zhang JJ, Wang H, Xuan JR, Chia RWJ, Hasenberg T, Kang HW. Dependence of water content in calculus phantom during Q-switched Tm:YAG laser lithotripsy. In: Proceedings of SPIE. Vol. 8565. Photonic Therapeutics and Diagnostics IX. 856519. San Francisco, California, USA: SPIE; 2013.

[20] Mues AC, Teichman JMH, Knudsen BE, FRCSC. Quantification of Holmium:Yttrium aluminum garnet optical tip degradation. Journal of Endourology. 2009;**23**(9):1425-1428

[21] Marks AJ, Mues AC, Knudsen BE, Teichman JMH. Holmium:Yttrium-aluminum-garnet lithotripsy proximal fibre failures from laser and fibre mismatch. Urology. 2008;**71**(6): 1049-1051

[22] Knudsen BE, Pedro R, Hinck B, Monga M. Durability of reusable holmium:YAG laser fibres: A multicenter study. The Journal of Urology. 2011;**185**:160-163

[23] Patel AP, Knudsen BE. Optimizing use of the Holmium:YAG laser for surgical management of urinary lithiasis. Current Urology Reports. 2014;**15**:397-404

[24] Manenkov AA. Fundamental mechanisms of laser-induced damage in optical materials: Today's state of understanding and problems. Optical Engineering. 2014;**53**(1):010901-1-7

[25] Kang HW, Lee H, Teichman JM, Oh J, Kim J, Welch AJ. Dependence of calculus retropulsion on pulse duration during Ho: YAG laser lithotripsy. Lasers in Surgery and Medicine. 2006;**38**:762-772

[26] Kuznetsov LI. Recoil momentum at a solid surface during developed laser ablation. Quantum Electronics. 1993;**23**:1035-1038

[27] Foth HJ, Meyer D, Stockel T. Side effects of laser tissue interaction studied by laser Doppler vibrometry. Proceedings of SPIE. 2000;**4072**:392-400

[28] White MD, Moran ME, Calvano CJ, Borhan-Manesh A, Mehlhaff BA. Evaluation of retropulsion caused by Holmium:YAG laser with various power settings and fibres. Journal of Endourology. 1998;12:183-186

[29] Lee H, Ryan RT, Kim JH, Choi B, Arakeri NV, Teichman JMH, Welch A. Dependence of calculus retropulsion dynamics on fiber size and radiant exposure during Ho:YAG lithotripsy. Journal of Biomedical Engineering. 2004;**126**:507-515

[30] Eisner BH, Pengune W, Stoller ML. Use of an antiretropulsion device to prevent stone retropulsion significantly increases the efficiency of pneumatic lithotripsy: An in vitro study. BM International 2009;**104**:858-861

[31] Robinson M, Teichman JMH. Laser lithotripsy retropulsion varies with stone mass. European Urology Supplements. 2013;**12**:e1063

[32] Finley DS, Petersen J, Abdelshehid C, Ahlering M, Chou D, Borin J, Eichel L, McDougall E, Clayman RV. Effect of Holmium:YAG laser pulse width on lithotripsy retropulsion in vitro. Journal of Endourology. 2005;**19**:1041-1044

[33] Lee HJ, Box GN, Abraham JB, Deane LA, Elchico ER, Eisner BFI, McDougall EM, Clayman RV. In vitro evaluation of nitinol urological retrieval coil and ureteral occlusion device: Retropulsion and Holmium laser fragmentation efficiency. Journal of Urology. 2008;**180**(3):969-973

[34] Marguet CG, Sung IC, Springhart WP, L'Esperance JO, Zhou S, Zhong P, Albala DM, Preminger GM. In vitro comparison of stone retropulsion and fragmentation of the frequency doubled, double pulse Nd:YAG laser and the Holmium:YAG laser. Journal of Urology. 2005;**173**(5):1797-1800

[35] Safer M, Watterson JD, Wollin TA, Nott L, Razvi H. Denstedt JD. Holmium:YAG laser lithotripsy for upper urinary tract calculi in 598 patients. Journal of Urology. 2002;**167**(1):31-34

[36] Cheung MC, Lee F, Yip SK, Tarn PC. Outpatient Holmium laser lithotripsy using semi-rigid ureteroscope. Is the treatment outcome affected by stone load? European Urology. 2001;**39**(6):702-708

[37] Lee Ryan RT, Teichman JM, Kim J, Choi B, Arakeri NV. Welch AJ Stone retropulsion during Holmium:YAG lithotripsy. Journal of Urology. 2003;**169**(3):88I-885

[38] Rajabhandharaks D, Kang HW. Short-pulsed Tm:YAG laser lithotripsy: Comparative study on ablation performance with conventional Ho: YAG laser. In: SPIE Photonics West BIOS Conference 8207B-47, Session 4: Therapeutics and Diagnostics in Urology: Lasers, Robotics, Minimally Invasive, and Advanced Biomedical Devices. San Francisco, California, USA: SPIE; 2012.

[39] Sroka R, Haseke N, Pongratz T, Hecht V, Tilld D, Stief CG, Bader MJ. In vitro investigations of repulsion during laser lithotripsy using a pendulum set-up. Lasers in Medical Science. 2012;**27**:637-643

[40] Carey RI, Kyle CC, Carey DL, Leveillee RJ. Preparation of artificial kidney stones of reproducible size, shape, and mass by precision injection molding. Journal of Endourology. 2008;**22**(1):127-131

[41] Delvecchio FC, Auge BK, Brizuela RM, Weizer AZ, Zhong P, Preminger GM. In vitro analysis of stone fragmentation ability of the FREDDY Laser. Journal of Endourology. 2004;**17**(3):177-179

[42] Vassar GJ, Chan KF, Teichman JMH, Glickman RD, Weintraub ST, Pfefer TJ, Welch AJ. Holmium:YAG lithotripsy: Photothermal mechanism. Journal of Endourology. 1999;**13**(3): 181-190

[43] Wieliczka David M, Shengshan W, Querry Marvin R. Wedge shaped cell for highly absorbent liquids: Infrared optical constants of water. Applied Optics. 1989;**28**(9): 1714-1719

[44] Blackmon RL, Irby PB, Fried NM. Comparison of Holmium:YAG and thulium fibre laserlithotripsy: Ablation thresholds, ablation rates, and retropulsion effects. Journal of Biomedical Optics. 2011;**16**:071403

Chapter 5

Extracorporeal Shock Wave Therapy: Non-Urological Indications and Recent Trends

Noha Maraie, Omar Mohammed Osman and
Hosni Khairy Salem

Additional information is available at the end of the chapter

http://dx.doi.org/10.5772/intechopen.69482

Abstract

Extracorporeal shockwave lithotripsy (ESWL) was introduced in 1980 as the preferred tool by the urologist for the treatment of renal stones and or upper ureteral stones. ESWL is minimally invasive procedures, exposes patients to fewer anesthesias, and has equivalent stone-free rates comparable to open surgery and endourology interventions for the treatment of renal stones. Urolithiasis is not the only application for extracorporeal shock waves but there are also other applications for it. Extracorporeal shock wave is used for the treatment of gall bladder stones, common bile duct stone clearance, pancreatic calculi, salivary stones, erectile dysfunction, and refractory angina pectoris chronic wound healing. This chapter gives full review about ESWL as minimally invasive procedures in the following items: (i) ESWL l in treatment of gall stones; (ii) ESWL for common bile duct (CBD) stones; (iii) ESWL for pancreatic stones associated with pancreatic pseudo cysts and chronic pancreatitis; (iv) ESWL in the treatment of salivary stones; (v) ESWL in the treatment of erectile dysfunction (ED); (vi) Cardiac shock wave therapy (ESWL) in treatment of refractory angina (RA); (vii) ESWL and chronic wound healing; (viii) Recent trends in extracorporeal shockwave lithotripsy (ESWL); (ix) Post ESWL complementary therapy; and (x) The future of ESWL in the year 2038.

Keywords: extracorporeal shock wave therapy (ESWT), extracorporeal shock wave lithotripsy (ESWL), gall stones, biliary stones, lithiasis, pancreatic stones, chronic pancreatitis, salivary stones, cardiac shock wave therapy (CSWT), erectile dysfunction, chronic wounds, healing, diabetic foot

1. Introduction

Shock waves are single high amplitude sound waves produced by electrohydraulic, piezoelectric or electromagnetic methods that are transmitted into tissues with sudden rise from low pressure to its highest pressure at wave front followed by lower tensile amplitude [1]. The international society for medical shock wave treatment [2] defines shock waves as sonic pulse characterized by high peak pressure (500 bar), short life cycle (10 ms), fast pressure rise (<10 ns) and a wide frequency spectrum. The shock waves are condensed at a zone of highest energy concentration in the targeted area within the treated tissues. The most important effects of shock waves are reflection with pressure and tension powers at levels of different resistance and the production of cavitation bubbles in liquids. These bubbles collapse and produce local shear forces by high velocity liquid streams (so-called jet stream) [1, 3, 4]. The introduction of ESWL during the early 1980s markedly changed the management of urinary tract stones, and during the last two decades, the development of new techniques of ESWL has changed completely the way of treatment of patients with renal stones [5]. ESWL was first successfully used in children in 1986 [6], and now, it is the first-line treatment of pediatric renal stones [7, 8]. Urolithiasis is not the only application for extracorporeal shock waves, but there are also other applications for it. Extracorporeal shock wave is used for the treatment of gall bladder stones [9], common bile duct stone clearance [10], pancreatic calculi [11, 12], salivary stones [13, 14], erectile dysfunction [15, 16], refractory angina pectoris [17, 18], and chronic wound healing [19, 20].

2. ESWL in treatment of gallstones

When ESWL was first used for gall stone lithotripsy, it was combined with bile acid therapy, which was only effective against non-calcified cholesterol stones. That is the reason why ESWL was only used against these types of stones [9]. However, some recent studies have proven that ESWL combined with bile acid therapy showed no significant improvement in gall stone clearance in comparison to ESWL alone [21, 22].

2.1. Efficiency of ESWL in comparison with cholecystectomy (CC)

Being minimally invasive, ESWL was preferred by patients and doctors to be used for gall stone clearance in contrast to surgery. However, cholecystectomy has proven less recurrence rates for gall stone development than ESWL [9].

On the other hand, a randomized, prospective study by Nicholl et al. [23] stated that both ESWL and CC groups had similar results regarding the 1-year health status following treatment. Moreover, the ESWL group health status was improved within 2 weeks in contrast to that of CC group that was improved in 5 weeks.

2.2. Future of ESWL in gall stones treatment

The lack of sufficient studies for the optimal application of ESWL in patients with gall stones hindered the Food and Drug Administration (FDA) approval for its use for gall stone lithotripsy.

However, this did not prevent several medical centers in Europe and Asia to use it for gall stone treatment on a constant rate [9].

3. ESWL for common bile duct (CBD) stones

Several studies reported the use of extracorporeal shockwave lithotripsy for common bile duct stones. As an instance, Tandan and Reddy [10] applied a certain protocol using ESWL for large CBD stones in their institute (Asian Institute of Gastroenterology, India). This protocol stated the start with endoscopic retrograde cholangiopancreatography (ERCP) as an initial procedure with placement of a nasobiliary tube to opacity the calculi to bath them in saline and to facilitate their targeting. This was followed by ESWL till the calculi were fragmented to a diameter less than 5 cm. Finally, ERCP is performed using a balloon or a basket to clear the CBD, and stenting was done only if indicated.

ESWL was indicated in all cases with large CBD stones with failure of their extraction by using the routine techniques; sphincterotomy followed by basket or balloon traw [10].

Tandan and Reddy reported some complications following the use of ESWL, including skin ecchymosis, pain at the site of administration, abdominal pain, occasional fever and hematobilia [10].

These complications can be reduced using a third-generation lithotripter with more accurate targeting and reduced patients' movements [24, 25].

4. ESWL for pancreatic stones associated with pancreatic pseudo cysts and chronic pancreatitis

A prospective study, by Li et al. [11], was performed on chronic pancreatitis patients with at least one stone in the main pancreatic duct of less than 5 mm in diameter. A total of 849 patients were divided into two groups: the case group was 59 patients with pancreatic stones and pancreatic pseudocysts (PPC) and the control group was 790 patients with pancreatic stones only. Following 116 ESWL sessions, 10.17% of patients in the PPC group showed complete stone clearance. Partial stone clearance occurred in 15.25% of patients. When ESWL was followed by ERCP, these percentages were raised to 67.24 and 20.69%, respectively. The authors concluded that ESWL—when followed by ERCP—was a successful strategy for lysis of pancreatic stones and regression of pancreatic pseudo cysts.

On the contrary, a retrospective study done by Vaysse et al. [12] has found that ESWL—as a sole treatment—was proven a safe and effective treatment for patients with obstructing stones in the main pancreatic duct. There was no need for adjuvant ERCP that showed no additional benefit. It was done on 146 patients with pancreatic duct stones resulting in chronic or recurrent acute pancreatitis. Only 132 patients continued to follow-up at 6-month period. About 69% of patients received adjuvant ERCP. At the end of 6 months, 76% of patients achieved successful treatment in the form of no need for analgesia, no acute pancreatitis or no need for surgical treatment for chronic pancreatitis. There were no significant differences in success rates between patients who received ESWL alone and those who received adjuvant ERCP.

5. ESWL in the treatment of salivary stones

ESWL sources used for salivary stones lithotripsy are either the electromagnetic source or the piezoelectric source. The electromagnetic shock wave source is more commonly used for being minimally invasive without need for anesthesia, so it can be done as an outpatient practice [26, 27]. Capaccio et al. [13] have done a prospective study on 415 patients on two groups in two time periods. Both groups received ESWL via an electromagnetic device that was preceded by ultrasonography (US) for localizing the stones. Follow-up was done using ultrasonography at 1 week, then at 1, 3, 6 and 12 months after ESWL application. Complete stone clearance percentages were generally higher in patients with parotid duct stones (group A: 69.3% and group B:68.8%) than in those with submandibular duct stones (group A: 35.9% and group B: 48.8%). However, with US follow-up, some residual submandibular and parotid dust stones were observed. Post-ESWL procedures to remove the symptomatic residual stones included sialendoscopy or transoral removal of stones. This proved that ESWL achieves good results for salivary stones especially parotid duct stones with small diameters.

In another retrospective study by Schmitz et al. [14], 31% of patients reached total stone clearance, and in 55% of patients, the treatment was partially successful with asymptomatic residual stone identified using US. Failure of treatment occurred in 14% of cases.

In spite of being non-invasive efficient alternative to surgery in management of sialadenitis, ESWL is contraindicated in the following cases: acute sialadenitis, gingivitis, pregnancy, bleeding disorders and calculi that cannot be detected using US. Relative contraindications include patients with cardiovascular diseases or artificial pace makers [13, 14].

6. ESWT in the treatment of erectile dysfunction (ED)

Several trials studied the efficacy of ESWT in the treatment of ED. Clavijo et al published a systematic review and meta-analysis of seven randomized clinical trials with 602 patients with vascular ED [15]. The seven studies used low-intensity shockwave therapy (Li-ESWT) for ED and used the erectile function domain of the International Index of Erectile Function (IIEF-EF) to assess the response to treatment. The IIEF-EF is a validated questionnaire that includes six questions about erectile frequency, firmness, penetration ability, frequency of maintenance, ability to maintain erection and erectile confidence on a scale of zero to five [28]. The difference in IIEF-EF score pooled change was measured in patients with ED treated with Li-ESWT and compared to that measured in patients treated with sham therapy. The IIEF-EF score in ESWL group was 6.40 points compared to the sham group which was 1.65 [15].

Another systematic review and meta-analysis by Fojecki et al. [16] included four studies that also used IIEF questionnaire, in addition to erectile hardness scale (EHS) to assess the success of treatment. One study of the four also examined the penile hemodialysis as an indicator for erectile dysfunction [29]. All of them compared ESWT to sham therapy. Three out of the four studies showed positive effect of ESWT on EHS scale compared to sham group. Only one study reported negative effect of ESWT on both EHS scale and IIEF score [30]. Hence, the effect of ESWT on ED is still inconclusive, although according to EHS scale, it is proven to have some potential in the treatment of ED [16].

7. Cardiac shock wave therapy (CSWT) in treatment of refractory angina (RA)

Cardiac shock wave therapy (CSWT)—which is also known as extracorporeal shockwave myocardial revascularization (ESMR)—represents a recent option for the treatment of refractory angina [17, 18]. Alunni et al. [17] performed a prospective case-control study over 6 months. They studied the efficacy of ESMR on cardiac perfusion in 72 patients with refractory angina (RA), 43 patients in the ESMR group and 29 in the control group (did not receive ESMR). They were compared at baseline and 6 months following ESMR therapy as regarding angina class score (CCS class score), the need for nitroglycerin consumption and the rate of hospitalization. Significant improvement in the patients' conditions occurred. Angina class score (CCS) improved in the ESMR group with an average of 1.33 versus 1.92 in the control group. Nitroglycerin consumption was lowered (20% in ESMR group versus 44.8% in control group) as well as the significant reduction in the rates of hospitalization (13.9% in the ESMR group versus 37.9% in the control group).

Vainer et al. [18] also applied cardiac shockwave therapy on the ischemic myocardial areas of 33 patients with end-stage coronary artery disease, chronic angina and reversible ischemia on myocardial scintigraphy. Patients were followed up after 1 and 4 months from the last CSWT session and assessed using CCS class score, their need for nitrate consumption, cardiac magnetic resonance imaging and myocardial scintigraphy. Follow-up showed an improvement in CCS score to drop from class III to class II, reduction in sublingual nitrate consumption from 10 times to twice per week, and myocardial scintigraphy showed improved myocardial perfusion. In conclusion, CSWT has proven to be an efficient non-invasive therapeutic option for patients with refractory angina.

8. ESWT and chronic wound healing

A recent systematic review done by Omar et al. [19] included 11 studies about the role of ESWT in the treatment of chronic wounds of lower limbs. A total of 925 patients were enrolled. About 85% of them received ESWT, and 15% represented the control group. Chronic wounds included diabetic foot ulcers (39.6%), traumatic wounds (20.3%), venous leg ulcers (12%) and others as pressure ulcers, acute burns, arterial leg ulcers, disturbed wound healing and surgical wounds. Several parameters were used to assess the rate and quality of wound healing. They include time to healing, reduction of wound surface area and tissue viability using laser Doppler perfusion imaging to measure the blood flow perfusion rate.

One of the included studies was done by the same author [20] as a single-blinded randomized controlled trial on the effect of ESWT in the treatment of chronic diabetic foot ulcers. They used almost the same parameters in measuring the rate of ulcers healing in addition to wound bed preparation. Standardized wound care was given, including wound debridement, blood-glucose control agents and special footwear to minimize the pressure. 20 weeks following the last ESWT session, 54% of ESWT group had completely healed ulcers versus 28.5% in the control group. There was significant reduction in the healing time with an average of 664.5 days in ESWT group versus 81.17 days in the control group.

The complications reported included pain, itching, infection, pigmentation and skin irritation. However, these complications were self-limiting and resolved in 5–7 days [19]. That is the reason why ESWT is recommended as an adjunctive therapy alongside with the standard wound care program [19, 20].

9. Recent trends in extracorporeal shockwave lithotripsy (ESWL)

The large number of patient treated by SWL in the past 25 years gives an important information about indications, contraindications, adverse effects of the procedures and the required development to improve the techniques of SWL for better treatment and less side effects [31]. Krambeck et al. [32] found that HTN incidence was significantly correlated with bilateral procedures done by using a Dornier HM3 lithotripter, while DM was correlated with shock wave number and frequency. The author postulate that occurrence of DM and HTN may be due to unobserved microtrauma on the pancreas and the kidney. Chew et al. [33] compared the incidence of DM and HTN in patient treated with an unmodified lithotripter HM3 (USWL) and second-generation modified HM3 lithotripter (MSWL); they found that there was no association between lithotripter and development of either DM or HTN in multivariate analysis and they suggest that the prevalence of DM and HTN in patient with renal stones is due to the presence of metabolic syndrome. Where there is increasing evidence, the patient with renal stones get HTN and DM and vice versa through this syndrome. Lee et al. [34] introduced that SWL treatment at frequency of 60 shocks/min gave better outcome compared with SWL at 120 shocks/min. On the other hand, pretreatment did not impact renal injury. Salem et al. compared slow and fast shock wave frequency, delivery rates in disintegrating pediatric renal stones smaller than 20 mm and the impact on stone clearance. Terms of comparison include treatment success, anesthesia time, secondary procedures, cost and efficiency quotient. They found that slow delivery rate of SWL has better stone clearance results than fast delivery rate [5]. Mazzucchi et al. [35] found no significant differences in the stone-free rate and complications development by reducing the total number of impulses from 4000 to 3000 and the frequency from

90 to 60 impulses/min. Vakalopoulos [36] developed a mathematical model to predict ESWL outcomes where predictive equations can be generated for different lithotripters. Wiesenthal et al. [37] developed a remarkable nomogram to predict the outcomes of renal and ureteral stone SWL treatment dependent on patient and stone factors. The risk of SWL failure is significantly related to increase radio density both in vivo and in vitro; cysteine, calcium oxalate, monohydrate and brushite stones are less liable to be treated by SWL [38, 39]. Salem et al. [40] conducted a prospective randomized trial over 200 patients comparing the SWL and semi rigid ureteroscopy for management of proximal ureteral calculi. He found that URS has higher free stone rate than SWL but more adverse effects so SWL should be the first-line treatment for proximal ureteral calculi of size < 1 cm. The introduction of second- and third-generation lithotripter not improves the stone-free rate or decreases the number of operations needed, but they have less anesthesia and minimal tissue injury [41, 42].

10. Post-ESWL complementary therapy

Micali and coworkers [43, 44] found the use of *Phyllanthus niruri* (a plant belonging to the euphorbiaceae family used in Brazilian folk medicine by patients with urolithiasis) with SWL lower calyx stone expulsion.

Also Micali [45] and Zheng et al. [46] found that the use of nifedipine and tamsulosin, both associated with ketoprofen after SWL of ureteral stones, increases stone-free rate for proximal and middle ureter (85.7% vs 51.7%) and distal ureter (82.1% vs 57.1%).

11. The future of ESWL in the year 2038

Understanding all effects of ESWL will lead to reliable production of <2 mm as sized reduction of the stones instead of fragmentation. This will result in a sawing back to non-touch shock wave lithotripter due to better shock wave generators with larger focal zones, respiratory regulated hit control based on color duplex ultrasound and computer-assisted shock wave navigation adapted to the individual anatomy. All will lead to increasing the quality of stone disintegration with almost complete pulverization of the stone, and these techniques can be applying without anesthesia producing no side effects [47].

Author details

Noha Maraie, Omar Mohammed Osman and Hosni Khairy Salem*

*Address all correspondence to: dr_hosni@yahoo.com

Faculty of Medicine, Cairo University, Cairo, Egypt

References

[1] Gerdesmeyer L, Maier M, Haake M, Schmitz C. Physical-technical principles of extracorporeal shockwave therapy (ESWT). Der Orthopade. Jul 2002;**31**(7):610-617

[2] (www.ismst.com)

[3] .Delius M, Ueberle F, Eisenmenger W. Extracorporeal shock waves act by shock wave-gas bubble interaction. Ultrasound in Medicine & Biology. Sep 1998 **30;24**(7):1055-1059

[4] Zelle BA, Gollwitzer H, Zlowodzki M, Bühren V. Extracorporeal shock wave therapy: current evidence. Journal of Orthopaedic Trauma. 1st Mar 2010;**24**:S66-S70

[5] Salem HK, Fathy H, ElFayoumy H, Aly H, Ghonium A, Mohsen MA, Hegazy AE. Slow vs rapid delivery rate shock wave lithotripsy for pediatric renal urolithiasis: A prospective randomized study. The Journal of Urology. 31 May 2014;**191**(5):1370-1374

[6] Newman DM, Coury T, Lingeman JE, Mertz JH, Mosbaugh PG, Steele RE, Knapp PM. Extracorporeal shock wave lithotripsy experience in children. The Journal of Urology. Jul 1986;**136**(1 Pt 2):238-240

[7] Muslumanoglu AY, Tefekli A, Sarilar O, Binbay M, Altunrende F, Ozkuvanci U. Extracorporeal shock wave lithotripsy as first line treatment alternative for urinary tract stones in children: A large scale retrospective analysis. The Journal of Urology. Dec 31 2003;**170**(6): 2405-2408

[8] Weir MJ, Tariq N, D'A. Honey RJ. Shockwave frequency affects fragmentation in a kidney stone model. Journal of Endourology. Sep 2000;**1;14**(7):547-550

[9] Mulagha E, Fromm H. Extracorporeal shock wave lithotripsy of gallstones revisited: Current status and future promises. Journal of Gastroenterology and Hepatology. Mar 10 2000;**15**(3):239-243

[10] Tandan M, Reddy DN. Extracorporeal shock wave lithotripsy for pancreatic and large common bile duct stones. World Journal of Gastroenterology. Oct 21 2011;**17**(39): 4365-4371

[11] BR Li, Liao Z, TT Du, B Ye, H Chen, JT Ji, ZH Zheng, JF Hao, SB Ning, D Wang, JH Lin. Extracorporeal shock wave lithotripsy is a safe and effective treatment for pancreatic stones coexisting with pancreatic pseudocysts. Gastrointestinal endoscopy. 31 Jul 2016;**84**(1):69-78

[12] Vaysse T, Boytchev I, Antoni G, Croix DS, Choury AD, Laurent V, Pelletier G, Buffet C, Bou-Farah R, Carbonnel F. Efficacy and safety of extracorporeal shock wave lithotripsy for chronic pancreatitis. Scandinavian Journal of Gastroenterology. 1 Nov 2016;**51**(11):1380-1385

[13] Capaccio P, Torretta S, Pignataro L. Extracorporeal lithotripsy techniques for salivary stones. Otolaryngologic Clinics of North America. 31 Dec 2009;**42**(6):1139-1159

[14] Schmitz S, Zengel P, Alvir I, Andratschke M, Berghaus A, Lang S. Long-term evaluation of extracorporeal shock wave lithotripsy in the treatment of salivary stones. The Journal of Laryngology & Otology. 2008;**122**(01):65-71

[15] Clavijo RI, Kohn TP, Kohn JR, Ramasamy R. Effects of low-intensity extracorporeal shockwave therapy on erectile dysfunction: A systematic review and meta-analysis. The Journal of Sexual Medicine. 13 Dec 2016

[16] Fojecki GL, Tiessen S, Osther PJ. Extracorporeal shock wave therapy (ESWT) in urology: A systematic review of outcome in Peyronie's disease, erectile dysfunction and chronic pelvic pain. World Journal of Urology. 1 Jan 2017;**35**(1):1-9

[17] Alunni G, Marra S, Meynet I, D'amico M, Elisa P, Fanelli A, Molinaro S, Garrone P, Deberardinis A, Campana M, Lerman A. The beneficial effect of extracorporeal shockwave myocardial revascularization in patients with refractory angina. Cardiovascular Revascularization Medicine. 28 Feb 2015;**16**(1):6-11

[18] Vainer J, Habets JH, Schalla S, Lousberg AH, Pont CD, Vöö SA, Brans BT, Hoorntje JC, Waltenberger J. Cardiac shockwave therapy in patients with chronic refractory angina pectoris. Netherlands Heart Journal. 1 May 2016;**24**(5):343-349

[19] Omar MT, Gwada RF, Shaheen AA, Saggini R. Extracorporeal shockwave therapy for the treatment of chronic wound of lower extremity: Current perspective and systematic review. International Wound Journal. 1 Feb 2017

[20] Omar MT, Alghadir A, Al-Wahhabi KK, Al-Askar AB. Efficacy of shock wave therapy on chronic diabetic foot ulcer: A single-blinded randomized controlled clinical trial. Diabetes Research and Clinical Practice. 31 Dec 2014;**106**(3):548-554

[21] Tsuchiya Y, Ishihara F, Kajiyama G et al. Repeated piezoelectric lithotripsy for gallstones with and without ursodeoxycholic acid dissolution: A multicenter study. Journal of Gastroenterology. 1995;**30**:768-774

[22] The East-Danish gallstone study group. Bile acid therapy versus placebo before and after extracorporeal shock wave lithotripsy of gallbladder stones. Alimentary Pharmacology & Therapeutics. 1996;**10**:651-657

[23] Nicholl JP, Brazier JE, Milner PC et al. Randomised controlled trial of cost-effectiveness of lithotripsy and open cholecystectomy as treatment for gallbladder stones. Lancet. 1992;**340**:801-807

[24] Tandan M, Reddy DN, Santosh D, Reddy V, Koppuju V, Lakhtakia S, Gupta R, Ramchandani M, Rao GV. Extracorporeal shock wave lithotripsy of large difficult common bile duct stones: Efficacy and analysis of factors that favor stone fragmentation. Journal of Gastroenterology and Hepatology 2009;**24**:1370-1374

[25] Tandan M, Reddy DN, Santosh D, Vinod K, Ramchandani M, Rajesh G, Rama K, Lakhtakia S, Banerjee R, Pratap N, Venkat Rao G. Extracorporeal shock wave lithotripsy and endotherapy for pancreatic calculi—a large single center experience. Indian Journal of Gastroenterology. 2010;**29**:143-148

[26] Chaussy C, Brendel W, Schmiedt E. Extracorporeally induced destruction of kidney stones by shock waves. Lancet. 1980;**2**(8207):1265-1268

[27] Ell C, Kerzel W, Schneider HT. et al. Piezoelectric lithotripsy: Stone disintegration and follow-up results in patients with symptomatic gallbladder stones. Gastroenterology. 1990;**99**(5):1439-1444

[28] Rosen RC, Riley A, Wagner G. et al. The international index of erectile function (IIEF): A multidimensional scale for assessment of erectile dysfunction. Urology. 1997;**49**:822-830

[29] Vardi Y, Appel B, Kilchevsky A, Gruenwald I (2012) Does low intensity extracorporeal shock wave therapy have a physiological effect on erectile function? Short-term results of a randomized, double-blind, sham controlled study. The Journal of Urology. **187**(5):1769-1775

[30] Yee CH, Chan ES, Hou SS, Ng CF. Extracorporeal shock–wave therapy in the treatment of erectile dysfunction: A prospective, randomized, double-blinded, placebo controlled study. International Journal of Urology. 2014;**21**(10):1041-1045

[31] Rosa M, Usai P, Miano R, Kim FJ, Agrò EF, Bove P, Micali S. Recent finding and new technologies in nephrolithiasis: A review of the recent literature. BMC Urology. 16 Feb 2013;**13**(1):10

[32] Krambeck AE, Gettman MT, Rohlinger AL, Lohse CM, Patterson DE, Segura JW. Diabetes mellitus and hypertension associated with shock wave lithotripsy of renal and proximal ureteral stones at 19 years of followup. The Journal of Urology. 31 May 2006;**175**(5):1742-1747

[33] Chew BH, Zavaglia B, Sutton C, Masson RK, Chan SH, Hamidizadeh R, Lee JK, Arsovska O, Rowley VA, Zwirewich C, Afshar K. Twenty-year prevalence of diabetes mellitus and hypertension in patients receiving shock-wave lithotripsy for urolithiasis. BJU International. 1 Feb 2012;**109**(3):444-449

[34] Lee JY, Moon YT. Evaluation of the optimal frequency of and pretreatment with shock waves in patients with renal stones. Korean Journal of Urology. 1 Nov 2011;**52**(11):776-781

[35] Mazzucchi E, Brito AH, Danilovic A, Ebaid GX, Chedid Neto E, Azevedo JR, Srougi M. Comparison between two shock wave regimens using frequencies of 60 and 90 impulses per minute for urinary stones. Clinics. 2010;**65**(10):961-965

[36] Vakalopoulos I. Development of a mathematical model to predict extracorporeal shock-wave lithotripsy outcome. Journal of Endourology. 1 Jun 2009;**23**(6):891-897

[37] Wiesenthal JD, Ghiculete D, Ray AA, Honey RJ, Pace KT. A clinical nomogram to predict the successful shock wave lithotripsy of renal and ureteral calculi. The Journal of Urology. 31 Aug 2011;**186**(2):556-562

[38] Leykamm L, Tiselius HG. Observations on intrarenal geometry of the lower-caliceal system in relation to clearance of stone fragments after extracorporeal shockwave lithotripsy. Journal of Endourology. 1 Apr 2007;**21**(4):386-392

[39] Ribeiro da Silva SF, Leite da Silva S, De Francesco Daher E, de Holanda Campos H, da Silva B, Antônio C. Composition of kidney stone fragments obtained after extracorporeal shock wave lithotripsy. Clinical Chemistry and Laboratory Medicine. 1 Mar 2010;**48**(3):403-404

[40] Salem HK. A prospective randomized study comparing shock wave lithotripsy and semirigid ureteroscopy for the management of proximal ureteral calculi. Urology. 31 Dec 2009;**74**(6):1216-1221

[41] Nabi G, Baldo O, Cartledge J, Cross W, Joyce AD, Lloyd SN. The impact of the Dornier compact delta lithotriptor on the management of primary ureteric calculi. European urology. 31 Oct 2003;**44**(4):482-486

[42] Lam JS, Greene TD, Gupta M. Treatment of proximal ureteral calculi: Holmium: YAG laser ureterolithotripsy versus extracorporeal shock wave lithotripsy. The Journal of urology. 31 May 2002;**167**(5):1972-1976

[43] Micali S, Grande M, Sighinolfi MC, Carne CD, Stefani SD, Bianchi G. Medical therapy of urolithiasis. Journal of Endourology. 1 Nov 2006;**20**(11):841-847

[44] Schuler TD, Shahani R, Honey RJ, Pace KT. Medical expulsive therapy as an adjunct to improve shockwave lithotripsy outcomes: A systematic review and meta-analysis. Journal of Endourology. 1 Mar 2009;**23**(3):387-393

[45] Micali S, Grande M, Sighinolfi MC, De Stefani S, Bianchi G. Efficacy of expulsive therapy using nifedipine or tamsulosin, both associated with ketoprofene, after shock wave lithotripsy of ureteral stones. Urological research. 1 Jun 2007;**35**(3):133-137

[46] Zheng S, Liu LR, Yuan HC, Wei Q. Tamsulosin as adjunctive treatment after shockwave lithotripsy in patients with upper urinary tract stones: A systematic review and meta-analysis. Scandinavian Journal of Urology and Nephrology. 1 Dec 2010;**44**(6):425-432

[47] Rassweiler J, Rassweiler MC, Kenngott H, Frede T, Michel MS, Alken P, Clayman R. The past, present and future of minimally invasive therapy in urology: A review and speculative outlook. Minimally Invasive Therapy & Allied Technologies. 1 Aug 2013;**22**(4):200-209